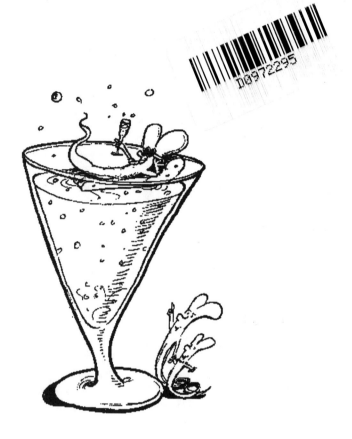

Drink to your health!

Who Is This Sproutman?

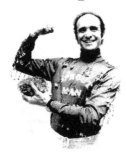

Steve Meyerowitz began his journey to better health in 1975 to correct a lifelong chronic condition of severe allergies and asthma. After two months of eating a living foods, vegetarian diet, his symptoms disappeared. After almost 20 years of disappointment with conventional medicine, Steve restored his health through his own program of purification, lifestyle adjustment, exercise, fasting, juicing and living foods.

Over the years, he has lived on and experimented with many so called "extreme" diet/lifestyles including, raw foods, fruitarianism, sprouts, dairy and flourless vegetarianism and fasting. In 1977, he was pronounced "Sproutman" by *Vegetarian Times Magazine* in a feature article that explored his innovative sprouting ideas and recipes.

After 10 years as a music and comedy entertainer, he made a complete lifestyle change for his health. In 1980, he opened *The Sprout House*, a "no-cooking school" in New York City. There, he began a formal program of teaching kitchen gardening and the preparation of gourmet sprouted and vegetarian foods. Steve has invented two home sprouters, the *Flax Sprout Bag* and *the Sprout House Tabletop Greenhouse* and founded the Sprout House, a company supplying juicers, growing kits and a full line of organic sprouting seeds.

Steve has been featured on the *Home Shopping Network, TV Food Network, in Prevention, Organic Gardening and Flower & Garden Magazines.* In 3 minutes on QVC, 953 people ordered his Cookbook and Tabletop Greenhouse.

Steve and his family, including three little sprouts, now live and breathe the fresher air of the Berkshire mountains.

J U I C E

FASTING

DETOXIFICATION

JUICE FASTING

and

DETOXIFICATION

Steve Meyerowitz

Sproutman ®

**Use the Healing Power of Fresh Juice
to Feel Young and Look Great**

The fastest way to restore your health

Illustrated by Michael Jon Parman

Distributed by
Book Publishing Company
PO Box 99, Summertown, TN 38483
888-260-8458. 931-964-3571. Fax 931-964-3518

SIXTH EDITION
Printed in the United States of America
ISBN 1-878736-65-5 Paperback

Publisher's Cataloging-in-Publication
(provided by Quality Books, Inc.)
Meyerowitz, Steve.
Juice fasting and detoxification : use the healing power of fresh juice to feel
young and look great / by Steve Meyerowitz ; illustrated by Michael Jon
Parman. –6th ed.
p. cm.
Includes bibliographical references and index.
Library of Congress Catalog Card Number: 99-90265
ISBN: 1-878736-65-5

1. Fasting–Health aspects. 2. Fruit juices–Health aspects. 3. Vegetable
juices–Health aspects. I. Title.

RM226.M49 1999   613.2'6
                      QBI99-333

Sproutman Publications
PO Box 1100, Great Barrington, MA 01230
413-528-5200, fax 413-528-5201
www.Sproutman.com   Email: Sproutman@Sproutman.com

Distributed by
Book Publishing Company
PO Box 99, Summertown, TN 38483
888-260-8458. 931-964-3571. Fax 931-964-3518
www.bookpubco.com e-mail: info@bookpubco.com

Cover art by Victor Zurbel, courtesy of
Omega Juicer, Harrisburg, PA. 800-633-3401
Cover Design by Keith Bona

Other Books

By Steve Meyerowitz
www.Sproutman.com

Water the Ultimate Cure
Discover Why Water is the Most Important Ingredient in your Diet and Find Out Which Water is Right for You. 2001.

Power Juices Super Drinks
Quick, Delicious Recipes to Reverse and Prevent Disease. 2000.

Wheatgrass Nature's Finest Medicine
The Complete Guide to Using Grass Foods & Juices to Revitalize Your Health. 1999.

Food Combining and Digestion
A Rational Approach to Combining What You Eat to Maximize Digestion and Health. 2002.

Sproutman's Kitchen Garden Cookbook
Sprout Breads, Cookies, Soups, Salads & 250 other Low Fat, Dairy Free Vegetarian Recipes. 1999.

Sprouts the Miracle Food
The Complete Guide to Sprouting. 1999.

Sproutman's "Turn the Dial" Sprout Chart
A Field Guide to Growing and Eating Sprouts. 1998.

Clinician's Complete Reference to Complementary/Alternative Medicine.
Steve Meyerowitz, co-author. Edited by Donald W. Novey, M.D. 2000.

Juice Fasting & Detoxification
Use the Healing Power of Fresh Juice to Feel Young and Look Great. 2002.

Table Of CONTENTS

HEALING

METHODS OF DETOXIFICATION

LOSING WEIGHT

PSYCHOLOGICAL EFFECTS OF FASTING

COMING OFF THE FAST

SPIRITUAL FASTING   117

REVIEW

HOW TO BUY A JUICER   129

RESOURCES

INDEX   145

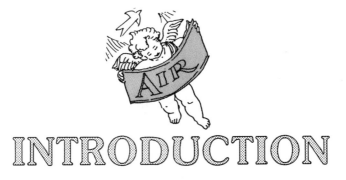

INTRODUCTION

*I tell you truly...Satan enter[ed] your bodies
which are the habitation of God. And he took in
his power all that he wished to steal: your breath,
your blood, your bones, your flesh, your bowels,
your eyes, and your ears. But by your fasting
and your prayer, you have called back the lord
of your body and his angels.*

-Jesus, Essene Gospel Of Peace

Our modern world is overflowing with food. Thanks to international commerce, food of every nationality, from every corner of the world can be found on our dinner plate. New inventions are coming out all the time with reconstituted gourmet meals in space age packaging, drinks contained in flexible tins bottles, gene-spliced cucumbers, and permanently preserved irradiated tomatoes, to mention a few. We are so involved with our food as a form of recreation, as a facilitator of our social life and as entertainment that we have forgotten the importance of *not* eating. Our fast-paced lifestyle along with modern commerce and advertising has blurred the relationship of food to our health. Yet, for all our technology and modern methods, we are plagued by a long list of contemporary diseases, many of them fatal, which modern medicine cannot cure. Lung cancer, colon cancer, heart disease, arteriosclerosis, high blood pressure and others were not prevalent 60 years ago and are directly linked to our diet and lifestyle.

Fasting is an age old cure that still works, even for modern ailments caused by our 20th century excesses. It is ironic that something so old works on problems so new and unfortunate that it is so ignored. But fasting is, in fact, our oldest health remedy. It is mentioned throughout the book of Exodus. Moses, Elijah and Jesus all fasted for up to 40 days. And Jesus speaks directly about fasting and diet in the *Essene Gospel of Peace*. (The latter differs from the New Testament in that it is a direct translation from the Aramaic text held in the library of the Vatican.) To this day Jews fast as a means of atonement. Christians fast during Lent. Moslems during Ramadan and Hindus fast routinely. Fasting was also advocated by Plato and Hippocrates and the Egyptians used it as a cure for syphilis. In modern times, the practice of therapeutic fasting was rekindled by a naturopathic physician, Dr. Isaac Jennings, in 1822.

What Is Fasting?

What fasting is, how it works and how you do it is the subject of this book. Fasting is simply a rest from food. It is uncanny that such a simple technique can work for such complex diseases. But it is true! The reason: our bodies are natural healers. Nature is both complex and sublimely simple. It works in minute mysterious ways that even modern science cannot fathom. Without obstacles in its way, our bodies will automatically seek health through the process of eliminating poisons and balancing chemistry. There is a vital force within us that can heal and when that vitality is not exhausted by physical activity, drained by the task of digestion or enervated by stress, it is available to heal. Fasting, essentially, promotes self-healing by casting off poisons. It is not so much a cure as it is an opportunity for rejuvenation, provided the essential organs have not been irreversibly damaged by disease or medical treatment.

The principle of fasting is straightforward: health restored through cleansing. Our bodies have a limited capacity to store and/or to eliminate non-digestible or foreign matter taken in through the diet. These materials, if left to circulate through the system, are antagonists to cells and organs and are collectively described as toxins. Our diets are replete with artificial colors, flavors, preservatives, pesticides, insecticides, rancid oils and other indigestible chemicals that overload our kidneys, bowels, skin, lungs and liver. As this toxic load accumulates from years of bad diet, air/water pollution, etc., it begins to interfere with normal functioning and our elimination becomes impaired. Natural hygienists theorize that this toxemia is the cause of "disease." A sick person's system is filled with poisons from the diet pollutants, lead, arsenic, medication, nicotine, cellular and metabolic waste products from wrongly combined foods, addiction to sweets, coffee, cigarettes and excessive eating--not to mention inadequate nutrition. You may get headaches upon waking, encrustation around the eyes, body odor, coated tongue, stuffy nose. The body discharges poisons in any way it can. A cold is merely a relief valve to relieve the lungs, blood, liver and lymphatic system of congestion. Stress combines with diet to compound the effects of this overload by impeding the normal flow of impulses. The nervous system can then no longer properly conduct the flow of vital energy to the various glands and organs. Lack of clarity, confusion, frustration and instability result. If ignored, these poisons become entrenched in the body and in time develop into chronic pathologies. Fasting reverses this toxic trend and liberates stored poisons.

The beauty of fasting lies in its simplicity. It is simply a practice of abstinence. Although some look askance and call it dangerous, their perspective has more to do with their fears and lack of knowledge. Fasting is largely a harmless practice that just about anyone can do. It is accepted and practiced in most countries as well as by the world's major religions. In contrast to today's exponentially expensive medical treatment with its maze of hospitals, doctors, laboratories, high-tech equipment, run-a-way health insurance premiums and out of control mal-practice litigation, fasting is something you can usually do yourself and it is free.

Today, health clubs, indoor sun tanning and body-building are in vogue. It seems that everybody wants a beautiful body. But they are designing their "look" in the same way they would buy furniture. Their focus is external. Fasters want beautiful bodies, too, but their focus is primarily internal.

Partial or Modified Fasts

In its strict definition, fasting is the total abstinence from all nourishment. A person who says they are on a juice fast or a fruit fast is actually describing a particular dietary regimen that limits their intake. But in either case, nutriment is being taken and that, in the strict sense, is not a fast. But there are numerous alternative diets and so we find new words entering our "health" vocabulary such as partial fasts, mono-diets, liquitarianism, etc.

A total fast, again, is one in which water alone is consumed or, at best, water with a squeeze of lemon. Juice fasting implies the taking of fruit or vegetable juices in addition to water. Fruit fasts are regimens in which only fruit is eaten. Mono-diets involve only one food per day. For example, an apple fast requires the eating of only apples for the day. They do not have to be only fruit. Macrobiotic followers often go on a brown rice mono-diet in which they eat only rice. Liquitarianism is a diet based solely on fiberless liquids. Juice is the primary drink on a liquitarian diet. However, a liquitarian regime may also include other liquids such as herbal teas, vegetable broths and almond or other nut milks, to name a few. But all must be strained, fiberless liquids.

All these modified fasts are described as fasts for a good reason. The word "fast" actually comes from the archaic Teutonic language *faestan* meaning "strict." These diets are indeed strict in the sense that they stick to a particular regimen, but because that regimen includes nourishment, they cannot be called fasts in the "strict" sense of the word. (Pun intended.)

But whatever the semantics, they have great value. All involve cleansing or balancing the body chemistry in some way. And, they provide a wonderful opportunity for those just starting out to "get their feet wet" if they lack sufficient knowledge or self-assuredness to enter a full-fledged fast. They are also a wonderful way of preparing the body and mind for a total fast, as we shall see, by providing a transition from a full diet to a full fast. More on these later.

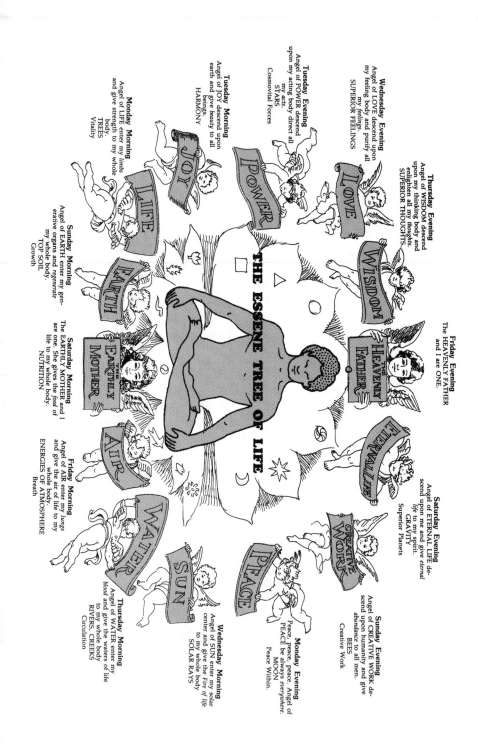

THE ESSENE TREE OF LIFE

Wednesday Evening
Angel of LOVE descend upon my feeling body and purify all my feelings.
SUPERIOR FEELINGS

Thursday Evening
Angel of WISDOM descend upon my thinking body and enlighten all my *thoughts*.
SUPERIOR THOUGHTS.

Tuesday Evening
Angel of POWER descend upon my acting body, direct all my *acts*.
STARS
Cosmovital Forces

Tuesday Morning
Angel of JOY descend upon earth and give *beauty* to all beings.
HARMONY

Monday Morning
Angel of LIFE enter my *limbs* and give strength to my whole body.
TREES
Vitality

Sunday Morning
Angel of EARTH enter my generative organs and regenerate my whole body.
TOP SOIL
Growth

Saturday Morning
The EARTHLY MOTHER and I are one. She gives the *food* of life to my whole body.
NUTRITION

Friday Evening
The HEAVENLY FATHER and I are ONE.

Saturday Evening
Angel of ETERNAL LIFE descend upon me and give *eternal life* to my spirit.
GRAVITY
Superior Planets

Sunday Evening
Angel of CREATIVE WORK descend upon humanity and give *abundance* to all men.
BEES
Creative Work

Monday Evening
Peace, peace, peace. Angel of PEACE be always *everywhere*.
Peace Within.

Friday Morning
Angel of AIR enter my lungs and give the air of life to my whole body
ENERGIES OF ATMOSPHERE
Breath

Thursday Morning
Angel of WATER enter my *blood* and give the waters of life to my whole body
RIVERS, CREEKS
Circulation

Wednesday Morning
Angel of SUN enter my solar center and give the *Fire of life* to my whole body
SOLAR RAYS

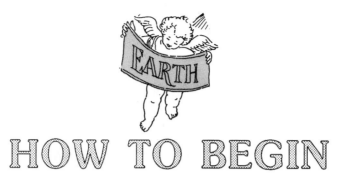

HOW TO BEGIN

Proper Motivation

In order to fast effectively, you have to be clear about what your intentions are. This may sound a bit facetious, but it is not uncommon for people to fast for the wrong reasons. Anorexia, for example, is a personality disorder in which people literally stop eating in order to conform to a distorted perception of themselves. They typically think they are overweight and stop eating even to the point of starvation. Bulimia is another eating disorder in which people binge on massive quantities of food only to regurgitate it all afterwards. Many waver between bingeing and purging and anorexia. Of course, they have a real desire to cleanse, but the constant fasting and bingeing cycle creates lots of physiological stresses and very little healing. Obviously, neither is a proper motivation for fasting.

There are other less drastic but still unhealthy reasons for fasting. There are those who fast or extend a fast simply for reasons of ego or image. Fasting can be an ego trip. If John can fast for 30 days then Jay wants to one-up him and fast for 40. Even if you feel it elevates your social position, fasting is not a vicarious practice. It must relate to your body and not to that of someone else. One's consciousness needs to be properly focused to gain the benefits fasting provides. Proper fasting begins with the purity of one's attitude towards it.

REASONS FOR FASTING

Social/Political Action   *Major Dental Work*
Spiritual/Personal Goals   *Healing The Body*
Personal Health Program   *Detoxification*
Break Food Addictions   *Weight Loss*

The most successful fasts begin with a great desire that comes from deep within and is solidly based in a physical or spiritual need. The predominant motivation for fasting is physical healing. Animals naturally fast when they are sick, and man/woman can benefit a lot from this practice. Instead of loading up the system with medicines, which interfere with the body's natural healing process or covering up the symptoms by sublimating the pain, fasting will cleanse the bloodstream, tissues and cells for deep, fundamental healing. Fasting does not cure as much as it rejuvenates. Although it may not be the preferred approach for every illness, there is a long list of ailments that have historically responded well to fasting. We use the word "historically" because fasting, to this day, is not recognized to be of legitimate therapeutic value by allopathic medicine. This being the case, it has not benefited from modern medicine's wealth of facilities and resources for research and experimentation. Traditionally, fasting has been used to improve a wide variety of ailments including some of the following:

Ailments Traditionally Treated with Fasting

Allergies	*Skin diseases*
Asthma	Acne
Bronchitis	Psoriasis
Hay fever	Ulcers
Hives	Boils
Rheumatism	
Obesity	*Digestive disorders*
Insomnia	Liver problems
Migraine headaches	Constipation
Inflammations	Gall stones
Arteriosclerosis	Diarrhea
High/low blood pressure	Tumors

Even if you do not have serious problems such as these, you may choose to fast purely for purposes of detoxification and health improvement. This is more a measure of prevention than a treatment for disease. Periodic fasting maintains an optimum level of functioning in the same way that cleaning your boiler once a year prevents breakdowns in the middle of the Winter. It is a matter of house cleaning. In addition, fasting increases energy and extends life. In a study on mice who were fasted every third day, their life span was increased by 40 percent.

Another major reason for fasting is weight loss. Fasting is probably the most rewarding of all the weight-loss regimens because the results come quickly and are visible. In fact, it is wonderful for all kinds of food addictions such as coffee, sweets, alcohol, smoke and other bad habits. (For more on weight loss, see p.97.)

Spirituality is the next most common motivation for fasting. The sheer task of living while not eating is a miracle to some. The mind clears, the whole body quiets and you are at once attuned to a different state of consciousness, one in which you hear, feel and think things that you would not ordinarily sense. Even if you are an agnostic, you will enjoy the feeling of well-being, like a joggers high, you get on a long fast. Fasting improves mental attitude and strengthens your discipline and resolve as you meet its personal challenge.

In recent times, fasting has been used as a tool for political and social change. Because our culture equates fasting with death, it has come to stand for a dramatic act of defiance that calls attention to the Faster and his cause. Some famous political fasters are Bobby Sands who fasted until his death; Dick Gregory who ran 15 miles on his 100th day juice fast; Andre Sakharov the Russian physicist and Mahatma Ghandi, the father of modern India.

Fasting has been used to heal gum problems and periodontal disease, but it is also a convenience during periods of painful dental work such as abscessed teeth, root canals and toothaches. No one enjoys food at these times and fasting helps to reduce the pain and promote healing.

Choosing The Right Time and Place

Now comes the big question--*When?* The success or failure of a fast may be determined by the chosen time. Fasting, remember, requires conservation of energy. It would be ill-advised to start a fast when physical, emotional or mental demands are being made on you. If you are an actress playing on Broadway and every night you have to exert yourself 100 percent, this would be the wrong time to fast. Every stressful day of your fast extends the time required to detoxify by one half day. That is, 15 days of fasting under stress would achieve the same amount of detoxification as a peaceful ten day fast. For fasting is not just a question of time, but is also one of energy. Yes, you are saving energy by not digesting food, but if you are spending it through emotional or mental stress, then it is not available for healing. The human body is a very intelligent machine. It will focus its attention wherever there are immediate needs. If there is an emotional crisis, the muscles will tighten, the adrenals will rev up, the heart will pump faster and the blood pressure will increase. No time for healing here. But if you are lying on a beach chaise on the shores of Waikiki sipping a lemonade, your body-machine will work on internal repair and house keeping. Dead cells and toxins will be eliminated. Liver cells will be rejuvenated. Small intestine and colon will purge themselves of unwanted matter, etc.

The idea of being on a beach is not a bad one. Vacation time is a good time to fast. The purpose of a vacation is to rest anyway, or at least it should be. One of the best vacations you can take for your body is a trip to a sunny health spa replete with mineral waters, steam baths, juice bar and surrounded by fresh air and fruit trees. If we put our annual health insurance premiums here each year, we would improve health as opposed to insuring against illness. But alas, our vacations usually involve the consumption of copious amounts of food which, in fact, is often one of the attractions. (For a solution, see p.29.)

If you are going on a Winter vacation, you probably should not fast even if you so desire. Unless it was January in the Bahamas, cold weather is not a faster's perfect environment. When you fast, you get cold. Food creates heat as measured in calories. The process of digestion is like combustion, it creates heat, as does exercise and activity in general. If you are inactive, however, you will get cold and without the calories of a normal diet, you will get cold more readily. The body consumes energy to create the heat necessary to compensate for and protect itself from the elements. On the other hand, weather that approximates normal body operating temperatures does not require additional energy to heat or cool itself. Warm sunshine is a wonderful healer. Your body is comfortable and the sun is relaxing and nourishing. That's right! When there is no other source of nourishment, your intelligent, magnificent body will transform light into vitamin D and energy. Just like solar panels, you can get a charge from the sun. But don't overdo it. If you are weak it will strengthen you, but if you are exhausted it will drain you. That is why the ocean figures into our little vacation scene. A cool ocean breeze moderates the temperature in addition to supplying moisture and negatively ionized air. Even the air is energizing! Ocean air fills you with its rich supply of nourishing oxygen and leaves you feeling strong.

Of course, you choose not to use vacation time. Alas, when else is there? Basically, the entire year is open to you. But please avoid times of stress, distraction and inconvenience. Visiting your family during Thanksgiving, for example, is a particularly poor time to fast. How do you break the news to your relatives? *"Don't take it personally, Mom, it's not your cooking. I just need to detoxify from all the other stuff you fed me over the years."* No matter how you try to express it, it just won't work. Try to complete your fasts well before Thanksgiving, birthdays, and other special occasions. (One exception: Some vegetarians prefer to fast on Thanksgiving as a statement of compassion for the condemned turkeys.)

Perhaps the one factor that supersedes all the others is your enthusiasm. If you have the passion, the esprit de corps, if you are "psyched," then it is the right time. Listen to your body. It will yearn for a fast when the time is right, whether Winter, Spring, Summer or Fall. If it is Winter, bundle up, stay warm and do whatever you need to protect yourself from the elements. Just remember, stress is the key. The more you insulate yourself from the elements and the vicissitudes of daily life, the less stress. The less you do, the quicker your fast will proceed and the less time it will take to achieve the desired results.

One more point. Remember our discussion of dental work. This is basically not an ideal time to fast because there are stresses involved and few of the other factors discussed are likely to apply. On the other hand, it is not a good time for eating either. Thus, as long as you are not going to enjoy your food, why not fast?

The Pre-Fast Diet

The purpose of the pre-fast diet is to prepare the body, physically and mentally, for the challenge of the fast. A typical pre-fast is from one to three days. You determine the length. All that is needed is enough time for the body to make the transition from solid food to juice. It is the perfect vehicle for those who have never fasted or who are hesitant about starting.

A typical pre-fast diet may consist of a day of cooked vegetables, salads, fruits and juices on the first day. Any food in these categories is acceptable, but it is still a limited diet because it excludes grains, breads, dairy, fish and flesh foods.

Day two is usually slightly more limited with only raw salads, fruits and juices. Day three might just be limited to fruits and juices. Each day is progressively more restricted up to the day of the fast. The fruits and vegetables are of course, eaten separately, e.g., fruits for lunch, vegetables for dinner. If time is limited and you are a seasoned faster, you may choose a one day pre-fast, which might turn out to be a day of salads or a day of fruits and juices. Always keep the juices and water in your pre-fast diet since they are the major elements of the actual fast.

Another type of pre-fast diet may be the mono-diet that we discussed earlier. A day of grapes would act as a strong detoxifying diet while still having the benefits of a solid food. Or you may choose a day of melons or apples or citrus. All are tremendously cleansing foods and would condition and prepare your body for the fast. Because of their detoxifying capacity, these foods may actually shorten a fast. If you wish to choose sprouts or lettuce that would be fine, but don't pick frankfurters! You must stick with the fruit and vegetable family and preferably eat them raw. Avoid nightshades--tomatoes, green peppers, potatoes and eggplant. A Macrobiotic brown rice diet would not be included because it is a grain. But then again, macrobiotics' do not fast.

Another type of pre-fast would be simply missing a meal or two. Take two or three days and skip dinner each day. Or, if it is easier for you, skip breakfast and lunch--your choice according to your schedule. You may find it easier to skip breakfast if you are running to work and have no time to enjoy it anyway. And you may be so busy at work that you could afford to overlook lunch.

Those of you who are sensitive to sugar should probably avoid the fruits. Even though these are wonderfully cleansing foods, if they affect your blood sugar levels, avoid them. Acid fruits may also be risky for some. Salads are the safest.

Pre-fasts are not fasts. Solid food is taken and there is no mental or physical disassociation with food. However, they are very beneficial in conditioning you mentally and physically and for those unable to fast, they may provide an opportunity to achieve some detoxification benefits.

Jumping In

Why not? If you already have fasting experience and self-confidence about what you are doing, then go ahead. It is like jumping in the ocean for a swim. If you have been there before, you know what to expect. It is going to be cold for the first few minutes. But it is nothing new, you have done this before. On the other hand, if you are unsure about yourself and do not swim often, you may choose to wade in slowly and adapt to the water little by little. This is the role of the pre-fast. But some personalities would prefer to dive in and get it over with no matter what. If you are one of these people, then be my guest. You are the captain of your ship and you know yourself best. You know your physical condition and you know if you have got the discipline to do it. Of course, a seasoned faster knows better than a beginner. As long as you have prepared yourself as best you know how, this is as good a way as any. If you've got the feeling, there is no time like the present to get started.

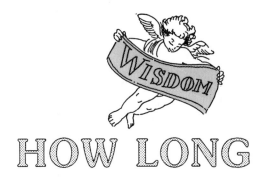

HOW LONG

To Fast

You probably already have some idea of how long you wish to fast. If someone suggested you fast for 30 days, your response may be a dramatic: "Oh, nooo...not me." Or it may be: "Yes, definitely if not longer..." In any case, you will always have a general sense of how long you plan to fast.

The duration of a fast depends on:

Fasting Experience
Physical Strength and Condition
Nature of Ailment If Any
Previous Diet
Mental Attitude
Level of Toxicity
Schedule of Work and Activities
Environment and Weather
Age

Short Fasts

Basically, there are two lengths of fasts, short and long. A short fast is anything under two weeks. Part of what defines a fast as short or long is its potential for harm. It is highly unlikely that a fast of two weeks or less will produce any irreparable damage, even if you do everything wrong. On the other hand, you could get yourself in trouble doing the wrong things for 30 days.

One Day A Week

Fasting one day a week is a wonderful practice which will repay you with a stronger immune system, longevity and vigor throughout your life. Give your system a break. Day in and day out you pile it in without a stop. The little workers inside your stomach are endlessly dealing with the new input you pile on, shoveling and sorting it in and out through dozens of feet of intestines and miles of circulatory highways. The workers are entitled to a day off. And you had better give it to them because you know what it feels like when they go on strike! Montezuma is not the only one who can take revenge.

What is a day off? It depends on which union you belong. Is it 24 hours or 36 hours? If you belong to the 24 hour union, start fasting Tuesday by missing dinner and return to eating Wednesday at dinner. You have missed three meals and fasted from approximately 6 p.m. to 6 p.m., 24 hours-- not a hard task, even for a beginner. If you keep yourself busy enough, you might not even notice it. Nevertheless, your body will, and it will be grateful. If you are in a 36 hour union, start fasting after dinner Tuesday, do not eat anything solid Wednesday, sleep tight Wednesday night and enjoy a "break-fast" Thursday morning. In this arrangement, you also miss three meals, but you include a sleep period. It is not so hard, because out of the 36 hours you spend 16 of them sleeping! That should help with your discipline. But it also helps with your detoxification. Sleep-time is when the body goes to work breaking down and eliminating wastes.

Anyone can do a one day fast. Consider the advantages of doing it once a week. If you fast one day a week, you will have fasted 52 days per year! Your body will thank you and you will live longer. There is always a day when you can schedule it. Pick one that does not conflict with other people's schedules. Avoid social occasions that require eating and entertainment. You do not want to be a sad sack at a Saturday night party and have to tell your friends you are fasting to improve your health! That just makes you seem odd. Although you may feel unique and want to tell the world about your experience, it is just your ego speaking. Fasting is not about that. Keep it to yourself. Fast on a day that does not involve too much stress, activity or interfere with other people's schedules. Attempt to keep the same day each week and vary only by one day if necessary. If your fasting day is Monday, perhaps a good choice after the weekend's excesses, extend it to Tuesday if you must because of occasional scheduling conflicts.

Another variation of the one-day fast is the *alternate day fast*. This is a 24 hour fast we described practiced every other day. Some people practice this method for purposes of weight loss. You get to eat, but you eat half as much with longer periods of rest for healing and waste removal. Just don't gorge yourself on the eating days. If you do, then this is not the fast for you.

Three Days and Longer

The next type of short fast is typically three days. This has the advantage of extending the fast after you have spent a day getting used to it. The first day, after all, is the hardest. It gets easier if you practice a pre-fast diet. But there is always a transition period and since you have made the effort, why not add a few more days and get a greater value for it? The three day fast amounts to a more sizable rest and if you have been pushing your gastrointestinal self too much, it will provide a much needed rest and recharging.

One day and three day fasts are wonderful for breaking the cycle of binges, cravings, sweets and other bad patterns or habits. They are especially good after overeating in general or at extenuated social events. Weddings are notorious for their temptation to cause us to overeat. And if you find yourself wobbling home after one, you might consider fasting soon thereafter. You will find that one or three days fasting returns the appetite, too, so you can really enjoy the pleasures of eating when you are doing it.

One Week - 10 Days - Two Weeks

These longer fasts, while still considered short, actually begin to develop the rhythm, feel and physiological response of a true fast. And they are no harder to do! If you are in tune with your fasting, that is to say, you feel good and are happy to continue, then it is no more effort to do 7, 10 or 14 days. (For more about being in "tune" with your fast see *Knowing When to Stop* p.105)

The hardest part of a fast is from days one through three when your body is making the transition from eating to fasting. That is both a physical process for your tummy and a mental and emotional chore for you. Physically, your body adjusts from transforming externally supplied calories into energy to using its own internally stored resources. Imagine an office worker whose desk is piled high with papers and projects. Each day more mail and more memos and more projects come in. He/she yearns for the day when the input would just stop so that they could catch up. If it would only stop, they would have enough work to keep them busy for several weeks. That is the way your system works. It has enough stored reserves to keep you nourished for a lot longer than most people would believe. Getting over the "hump" is the hardest work. It is like jogging beyond the 5 mile point. Then your body goes on automatic and it is remarkably easy. During the first three days, there is also that feeling of emptiness that always returns when you are constantly filling your stomach with bulk. That too, lapses. It is just a matter of readjustment.

While the one to three day fast allows your system to "catch up" or do general house cleaning, the seven to fourteen day fast affords deeper cellular elimination and repair. Let's face it, some people will never fast for 30 days. If a one or two week fast is all you can handle, then make the best of it. Fast at least once a year. Do it every Spring or Fall. Pick a time and be regular. After all, the effects of a long fast diminish with time. If you fasted 45 days 8 years ago, that has little consequence to your ongoing health program today. You must fast regularly just as eat regularly. An excellent program is a two week fast once per year.

Long Fasts

Fasts of over two weeks are generally considered long and, here, experience and guidance is recommended. Like any journey, one of the most important first steps is to remove fear of the unknown. Study, plan and consult. Make preliminary contact with health practitioners who are partial to fasting such as chiropractors, naturopaths, homeopaths, physical therapists, osteopaths or even naturally oriented physicians. They can be very helpful. A physical check up prior to a long fast is a must if a serious health problem is involved. Full experience, of course, can only be acquired by actual involvement.

Longer fasts afford deep cellular repair, elimination, and rejuvenation and are usually called for to help chronic conditions such as arthritis, asthma, arteriosclerosis, ulcers, psoriasis, tumors, hay fever, hive, migraines, rheumatism, obesity, high blood pressure, etc. These problems are deep seated, but it is not impossible for you to fast 30, 45, 60, 75 days or longer to heal yourself. Not all problems are fully resolved in this time. No matter how long the fast may seem to you, it is really quite brief in comparison to a lifetime of wrong living. In fact, many times a series of fasts are required to achieve complete wellness. A single long fast will certainly mitigate symptoms and reduce pain in most cases, and it makes the ongoing healing process more manageable for the body during the regular eating period. Long term fasters often feel "born again" and would readily trade 75 or even 100 days of food for these life saving results.

Chemical Changes During Fasting

Chemically speaking your fast is divided into three stages. The first few days of your fast is primarily devoted to body reorientation. Your system starts to change the pH of your stomach upward making it more alkaline. The stomach contracts and the digestive tract is cleansed. Here also you will experience the most dramatic weight loss. Water, minerals--especially sodium and potassium--and water soluble vitamins are heavily excreted in the early days. Protein loss is up to 75 grams per day in the beginning, while only 18-20 grams later. You may experience hunger, headaches, light headedness or sweating and you may urinate a lot. Bowel movements may come daily or never.

During the second phase, the liver starts to purge itself of its chemical and toxic load throwing off these poisons into the bloodstream for elimination. You may experience nausea, exhaustion, diarrhea, muscle aches, nervousness, shortness of breath, trembling...all the symptoms of a flu. Your tongue will coat, you may develop bad breath, body odor and/or skin eruptions. Basically, your body is battling the pollutants as if you had just consumed them. Poisons sting twice: once on the way in and again on the way out. They could be anything, illicit drugs, prescription medicines, food preservatives, artificial flavors, agricultural pesticides or the products of cooking or bad food combining. The process of natural healing often involves briefly getting worse before you get better.

During the third phase, deep tissue cleansing begins, blood toxins are removed and cellular ash and debris are flushed from the kidneys. The third phase combines some of the symptoms of the first two phases along with bursts of energy. Gradually you gain a total feeling of well being. This is the period of organ detoxification and regeneration. It's a mixed bag. You may experience euphoria or stress, irritability or improved mental attitude and self-esteem.

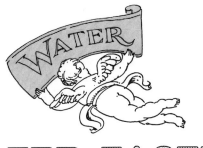

WATER FASTING

*Would that you could live on the fragrance of
the earth and like an air plant be sustained by
the light.*

--Kahil Gibran, The Prophet

Drinking only water is what most people think of when
they think of fasting. However, this kind of fast is not for
everyone. Water fasting is an arduous task that requires strict
control of the fast's conditions and circumstances.

Rest

Rest is the key word here. This means inactivity, no
stress, and ideally, a clean environment to rest in. Solitude
and silence are ideal if you can manage to secure such an
atmosphere. Keep to yourself. Avoid talking, listening to the
radio and TV. Do not drive (your reactions are slower).
Bathe in the sun. Do yoga. Lie in the grass and let nature
absorb the poisons in your body and balance your aura. Be
prepared for the unfolding of some of your psychic abilities.
Choose clean, fresh air by the seashore or on a mountain.

Fasting in general, and water fasting in particular, requires total submission to rest. It is a kind of human hibernation. What energy you have is directed toward the vital job of detoxification and cleansing.

REQUIREMENTS FOR A WATER FAST

Personal
Keep to yourself
Avoid TV and radio
Bathe in the sun
Lay on the grass
Do yoga
Plenty of fresh air
Lots of rest, No stress
Previous fasting experience
Read fasting or spiritual books

Environmental
No pollution
Seashore or Mountains
Forest or Countryside
Sub-tropical

Ordinarily, when you are not fasting, this process of breaking down and cleaning up (catabolism) goes on each night when you go to sleep. The fast, however, allows the perpetuation of these catabolic processes during the day. Ordinarily, catabolism is halted in the daytime due to activity and stress. Energy is directed into the muscles and digestive system. Muscular activity requires the removal of lactic acids, pyruvic acids and other by-products. Digestion, in turn, secretes fluids from glands. The nervous system collects and distributes signals. The liver catabolizes chemicals and disposes and neutralizes unusable matter and internal muscular activity takes place in the stomach and intestines. This is a lot of work for a body! And since you are not taking in the proper calories and nutrients needed for this kind of activity during a fast, your body is further strained and the fast can actually do more harm than good in this situation.

Speaking of activity, sexual activity should be avoided while fasting and until full strength is recovered. Sex redirects the amount of available energy to the sexual organs for stimulation. This is a setback to the fasting process and a stress on your whole system since the sexual organs are dormant and would need to be revitalized.

Let it be clear that this author is in favor of water fasting. But only for those who are so inclined who are willing to work within the limitations and able to provide the right conditions. If you are a water fasting person, you will know it. It is almost as if it is a biological decision. Juice fasting will repel you. You will automatically gravitate to and prefer just water. It is a preference that is automatic and apparent. If it is for you, then you will find it easy. If it is not, you will find it impossible. Most people, in today's fast paced world, prefer juice fasting or some other regime. In general, water fasting is best for healthy people who have lived naturally and want to improve their spiritual and physical well being. If you think this kind of fast is for you, attune your body first with a pre-fasting diet. Don't forget to drink plenty of water--at least the equivalent of one glass every hour.

Breatharianism

Breatharianism, as you may have guessed from the name, is the ultimate in fasting. Not only don't you take in any food, you don't take any water! What's left? Just air and sunshine and love. This kind of fasting definitely requires a pure non-polluted environment. Silence and solitude are also high on the list. Obviously, it is not for everyone, in fact, very few. But if you are inclined to dabble, first become a seasoned water faster and on your next water fast, take one day off and have no water. Just take one day if you want to experience breatharianism. But remember, caution is in order breatharianism is only for those who know they are ready. (See Spiritual Fasting p. 117.)

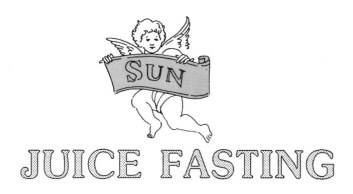

JUICE FASTING

Is It Fasting At All?

First of all let us set the record straight. Juice fasting is an inherent misnomer. Juice fasting is not a true fast but a liquitarian elimination diet. That's just terminology. The effect is that you are not eating solid food and you are losing weight and detoxifying. From here on, we will bend the traditional definition with the customary application and use the word "fast."

Why Juice Fasting?

Semantics aside, this is an ideal way for first timers to start and for experienced fasters to "work-along" while they detoxify. Unlike water fasting, juice fasting supplies calories and nutrition and thus protects you, at least partly, against the stresses of work and activity. In other words, you do not need to spend your vacation time fasting, you can do it while you work. I call this the "Big Apple Fast" because it maintains enough energy for you to work, almost at the normal pace, and protects you against the toxins and stresses of life in a polluted big city environment. Juices are concentrated nutritional elixirs that nourish you and provide the stamina you will need without necessitating much alteration of lifestyle.

Concentration and Assimilation

Nothing is more nutritious than juice. Imagine eating a meal of spinach, parsley, sprouts, tomatoes, lemon, celery, radishes, green pepper and cucumber. Ordinarily, considering the normal state of our digestive systems, we would be lucky to digest 70 percent of it. But once you extract the liquid portion of these vital foods, you can assimilate and absorb up to 99 percent of the food value even if you have weak digestion. In fact, the beauty of it is that it barely takes any digestive energy at all, which is why it is so suitable for fasting. This condensing of pounds of valuable foods into a single glass while simultaneously maximizing assimilation is what makes drinking juices special. Take carrots for example. It takes a pound of carrots to make a 10½ ounce drink of carrot juice...mmm, delicious. But could you consume that many carrots? Absolutely not! Yet all the enzymes, water soluble vitamins, minerals and trace elements in those carrots are extracted (assuming it is a quality juicing machine) and condensed into the glass of juice.

This is the whole concept behind a vitamin pill: a concentration of nutrients in a pill. But it is not the same thing. Vitamins involve several steps of processing along the journey from a fresh food into a tablet. Many of those steps may involve heat, which destroys or alters nutrients. Chemical solvents may also be involved. Or, of course, the nutrients may not even be natural at all but synthetic. Manufacturing tablets and capsules involves adding ingredients other than the active ingredient. These are called excipients. They can be anything from sweeteners, to stabilizers, coloring agents, fillers, talc, binders, etc. A far cry from a glass of fresh spinach! If you are trying to heal, choose live food: the juice of living plants.

Fiber

One more point. Many people wonder about the value of drinking juice after all the promotion and praise they have heard regarding whole foods. In other words, the fiber in carrots is healthy. Why eliminate it?

The promotion of whole foods is certainly a concept this author supports. Its origins date back to the removal of bran and germ from flour and the extraction of molasses from sugar, etc. However, these processes are vastly different, involving chemical solvents and the destruction of vital nutrients. In contrast, juice brings out the vital nutrients in foods and makes them more readily available for digestion. The fiber in carrots, for example, is indeed an important nutritional factor and they should be consumed whole and raw. But one does not have to exclude the other. Eat fresh carrots and other fresh vegetables and fruits. Think of your juices as supplements and as medicines. And when fasting, think of them as your meals.

TYPES OF
JUICES

A juice diet differs greatly from a water fast in that it encompasses a vast smorgasbord of tastes and flavors. You will never get bored on a juice fast. If fact you may be having such a good time you might start to wonder what exactly it is you are sacrificing!

Fresh Fruit Juices

Fasting aside, when most of us think of juice, we think of fruit juices. The most widely consumed juice in the world is orange juice with apple juice following as a close second. Grapefruit, grape, prune and cranberry are also on the hot-to-drink list. Tomato juice is very popular and although technically a fruit, it is not generally classified as fruit.

You can take fruit juices any time of day. They are good in the morning for breakfast, for lunch, or as an after-dinner snack. Think of your juices as meals. Have as much as you like. Typically, that is 8 ounces to 16 ounces, but not more than 20 ounces. Do not gorge yourself with juice just as you would not gorge yourself with food. On average, a 10 or 12 ounce serving is plenty.

Fruit juices should be mixed with other juices throughout the course of the day. One or two fruit juices per day should suffice. Some people prefer as little as possible or none. That is your choice and it should be guided by knowledge of your own health and condition such as blood sugar sensitivities.

Mixtures

You may also choose to mix your fruit juices together. There are several wonderful blends.

Apple & Pear
Apple, Pear & Pineapple
Orange & Grapefruit
Apple & Watermelon

Apple & Prune
Apple & Cranberry
Apple & Grape

Fruits, as a group, are basically cleansing foods. Their high water content flushes your digestive tract, your kidneys and purifies the bloodstream. Many fruits, particularly citrus, are strong solvents. Lemon is the strongest, followed by lime, pineapple and grapefruit. All have a purging effect on the liver and gall bladder. Pineapple contains the enzyme bromelain which encourages the secretion of hydrochloric acid and helps digest protein. Grape, although only a sub-acid fruit, is known as a powerful cleanser. You can get a sense of that if you ever make fresh grape juice. Using the natural seeded variety, it is necessary to dilute the juice with water before consuming it. Concord grapes are the strongest. Apples are also excellent intestinal brooms. They contain malic acid and galacturonic acid both of which help remove impurities and pectin which prevents the putrefaction of protein. They also act as a bulking agent gently pushing through the digestive tract and cleaning it along the way. Many people choose apples as a mono-diet for this reason. Cranberry is an excellent diuretic whose bitter taste is very healing to the kidneys. Watermelon juice is also a diuretic particularly if you juice the rind. And why not? Your juicing machine can turn this ordinarily inedible portion into fresh juice. Prune and apricot juice help to soften the bowels and instill movement.

Watch out for berries and oranges. Lots of people have allergies to berries and you do not want itchy eyes or skin when on a fast. Besides, these fruits supply relatively little juice. Any fruits not mentioned here are wide open territory for you to try. Avoid any that may stimulate potential allergies and those that are non-juicable.

The Unjuicables

Papaya	*Honeydew*
Coconut	*Peach*
Banana	*Plum/Prune*
Strawberry	*Apricot*
Cantaloupe	*Avocado*

What does this mean? Certainly you have had papaya juice, apple-banana, apple-strawberry, apple-apricot and pina-cola (pineapple-coconut) juice. Not so! These fruits are un-juicable meaning their pulp does not easily separate from their water. Take a banana, mash it up any way you can, then run it through your juicer. Does any water separate out? No! The same thing with the other fruits listed here. Then why the mystery? Papaya juice, for example, is a mis-nomer. It is not a juice at all. The manufacturers blend up the pulp of the papaya fruit and mix it with water or sweeteners or other fruits juices such as apple or grape. Apple-apricot juice is apricot pulp blended with apple juice. Berries do release some water, but the amount of strawberry, or blueberry juice released is so small that it would be very costly to sell quarts of it. So, juice makers add 70 to 80 percent apple or grape juice to their berry "juice" mixtures. These are not quite juices but juice with fruit pulp. Some labels will say so. In the case of papaya, or wherever water is added, the correct commercial appellation is papaya "drink." Read your labels. Coconut drink is coconut meat blended with water and sweetener. Coconut milk, however, is the natural sweet water that forms inside the coconut hull. This is delicious and perfect for a fast, but it is expensive and hard to store so you will only get it with a hammer and a knife.

Watermelon is a wonderful juicy fruit, but not so for the other melons. Cantaloupe and honeydew are too pulpy and do not yield a lot of juice. The juiced product is very viscous and contains virtually all the fiber of the original fruit. It is simply not an extract of the fruit and they are better eaten than juiced. Prune juice is also a misnomer. Try sticking some prunes through your juicer (and don't forget to remove the pits!). After your machine grunts, stumbles and snarls, you will see what I mean. Prune juice is made by soaking prunes, which are actually dried plums, and extracting their water by osmosis. It is simply an extract, not a juice. No dried fruits, such as raisins or figs, will make a "juice." But you can soak them and enjoy the flavors, sugars and nutrients that these foods release into the water. Just soak one cup of raisins in one quart of water for 8 to 10 hours. They are delicious and perfect for a fast. You can even get two soakings from one batch.

Pasteurized Juice vs. Fresh Juice

Don't get too excited about guzzling down delicious fruit juices unless you plan to make them yourself. Bottled juices must be pasteurized in order to have a shelf life. Of what significance is that? Pasteurized juices are boiled to sanitize these foods against bacteria and disease organisms. Unfortunately, enzymes and many vitamins are destroyed along with it. Your only source of nourishment is these juices and you cannot afford to drink enzyme-less and vitamin poor liquids. Do not be fooled by the delicious taste and interesting assortment of flavors. Though they taste good, they are basically dead foods. There is no live nutrition left--only sugar, flavor and water. Even the taste and color is no match against the fresh squeezed version. Which do you prefer--fresh squeezed orange juice or the store bought kind? If you like your orange juice fresh, you will really be amazed at the difference between fresh squeezed and bottled apple juice. Fresh apple juice is white--just like the color of the apple when you bite into it. Bottled apple juice is brown because vitamins have been oxidized upon contact with the air. Just exposing live nutrients to air and light is enough to destroy some of these fragile friends. Run your apples through your juicer machine and taste the difference. Notice the word "bottled." All juices sold in bottles are pasteurized, but juice is also sold in wax containers and plastic jugs. When apple juice is sold in plastic jugs, you will notice the term "cider" is used. Cider implies that the juice was not pasteurized and is just fresh squeezed. It is perishable and in fact you need to read the label carefully to make sure no preservatives are added. If you see the words "cider" on bottled apple juice, it is incorrect and misleading labelling. Manufacturers can get away with it because the terms have been used loosely for a long time and the regulatory agencies have not laid down strict definitions for them.

You can drink cider on your fast. It is fresh apple juice if you buy it in a jug. You can tell it is fresh because the jug will expand when the cider starts to ferment. Do not hesitate to squeeze those jugs! (Pun not intended.) If they are flexible, you have found freshly squeezed apple cider-- the best. If they are tight and swollen, you have already fermented cider and you should choose another jug. Wax containers also allow for expansion due to possible fermentation, but the vast majority of these containers have been pasteurized anyway. Fresh squeezed juice is almost always sold in plastic jugs because if they were packed in jars, the bottles could explode on the shelves.

Carrot Combos

Probably the most popular drink of the health movement is carrot juice. Years ago, there just wasn't any such thing. Now, it is the "in" thing. Juice bars and health stores have sprung up all around the country serving carrot juice and variations based on it. It has become such a commodity that it is even shipped across the country in refrigerated-freezer trucks to be sold as frozen juice in health food stores. In addition to its image as a healthful drink, now consumers have scientific verification of how beneficial it is to drink carrot juice. Cancer research has acclaimed beta-carotene, the form of vitamin-A in carrots, as a cancer-fighting nutrient.

But is carrot juice really that good? Yes and no. It is as good for you as carrots. But what about all the other wonderful vegetables around us. Spinach, parsley, beets, peppers, etc., are all nutritious. Carrot is by far the sweetest and some say the prettiest, but spinach has more protein and more vitamin A. But just a minute--let's not start a fight amongst our favorite vegetables! Why not just mix them all together. Such as:

Carrot Combos

CARROT
CARROT BEET
CARROT BEET GREEN PEPPER
CARROT BEET GREEN PEPPER CUCUMBER
CARROT BEET GREEN PEPPER CUCUMBER PARSLEY...OR

CARROT APPLE
CARROT APPLE ALFALFA SPROUTS
CARROT APPLE ALFALFA SPROUTS WATERMELON RIND
CARROT APPLE ALFALFA WATERMELON RIND GINGER

CARROT SPINACH
CARROT SPINACH CARROT TOPS
CARROT SPINACH CARROT TOPS ALOE VERA...OR...

CARROT CABBAGE...OR...
CARROT SWEET POTATO...OR...
CARROT CABBAGE PARSLEY...OR...
CARROT SUNFLOWER SPROUTS...AND MANY MORE...

How Much - How Often

Drink juice until your stomach is content. No harm can come from this except the experience of a full belly. The average juice serving is 10 ounces at a sitting. Sixteen ounces, however, is not unheard of especially if you are thirsty. Twenty and 25 ounces, however, are a lot and if you are drinking this much perhaps what your body is saying is that you really want to eat. How many times per day? Once or twice a day is average. But you don't have to stick to that. If it suits you, drink a carrot combo once every other day. After all, there are so many other wonderful drinks and juices to choose from.

Juice Sweet

If you love carrot combos, have more. Just remember that carrot juice is sweet and too many sweets are just as bad on a liquid fast as they are in solid food. That is the advantage behind the carrot combos. Carrots alone would be too sweet. You can actually get a toothache or a low blood sugar attack even on a juice fast. So be careful. Your body is more susceptible to blood sugar addictions without the influence of other solid foods. Mix your carrots with the other vegetables especially the green ones to moderate the sweetness or dilute with water. And that's not all. Mixing varies your nutritional intake and that is important on a fast. By the way, it is perfectly all right to drink sweet combos like carrot, beet, apple, watermelon rind, etc. There is always a time and place for such a drink and it all depends on you, your personal preference and disposition. But overdoing these sweet juices may lower your blood sugar levels and bring on cravings that would be detrimental to your health and the continuation of the fast.

What Proportions

How about proportions? Carrot always dominates. In a 10 ounce serving of carrot, beet, apple and watermelon rind, 5 ounces would be carrot, 1 ounce beet, 2 ounces apple and 2 ounces watermelon rind.

More Carrot Juice Combinations
Recipes in juice ounces per 12 oz drink

5 Carrot
2 Beet
2 Green Pepper
2 Cucumber
1 Parsley

7 Carrot
2 Parsley
2 Cucumber
1 Radish

7 Carrot
3 Spinach
1 Carrot Top
1 Aloe Vera

8 Carrot
1 Beet
1 Broccoli sprouts
2 Celery

5 Carrot
2 Apple
2½ Alfalfa Sprouts
2 Watermelon Rinds
½ Ginger

5 Carrot
2 Celery
1 Beet
2 Spinach
1 Cabbage
1 Green Pepper

8 Carrot
3 Celery
½ Cilantro
½ Garlic

6 Carrot
2 Spinach
2 Kale
2 Red Pepper

6 Carrot
3 Celery
1 Beet
2 Spinach

6 Carrot
2 Tomato
2 Celery
2 Spinach

7 Carrot
2 Spinach
1 Beet
2 Cabbage

6 Carrot
2 Parsley
2 Spinach
2 Kale

One Cup of
Carrot Juice

Calories	98.0	Cobalamin-B12	0.0mcg
Protein	2.32g	Folacin	9.40mcg
Carbohydrate	22.8g	Pantothenic	0.560mg
Dietary Fiber	3.34g	Vitamin C	21.0mg
Fat-Total	0.36g	Vitamin E	-.-iu
Fat-Saturated	0.066	Calcium	58.0mg
Fat-Mono	0.018g	Copper	0.114mg
Fat-Poly	0.174g	Iron	1.13mg
Cholesterol	0.0mg	Magnesium	34.6mg
Vit A-Carotene	6318.0iu	Phosphorus	102.0mg
Vit A-Preformed	0.0iu	Potassium	716.0mg
Thiamin-B1	0.226mg	Selenium	1.80Mcg
Riboflavin-B2	0.134mg	Sodium	72.0mg
Niacin-B3	0.946mg	Zinc	0.442mg
Pyridoxine-B6	0.532mg		

Weight is 246.0 grams or 8.68 ounces	
Water Content	219.0g
Calories from Protein:	9%
Calories from Carbohydrates:	88%
Calories from Fats:	3%
Polyunsaturated /Saturated fat Ratio	2.6:1
Sodium /Potassium Ratio	0.1:1
Calcium /Phosphorus Ratio	0.6:1

What's that? Carrots mixing with apples? It's true. Although we may not ordinarily mix fruits and vegetables because it is poor food combining, the combining rules for solid foods do not always hold for liquids. Remember, juices are mostly water and the versatility of mixing different liquids is much greater than that of solids. The main exception here is the mixing of acid fruit juices such as lemon, grapefruit or orange. Acids can curdle other liquids and with some exceptions are usually mixed among themselves. Some acids, by the way, such as the digestive enzyme malic acid in apples, can cross over the fruit/vegetable line even, to a degree, with solid foods. For this reason, you may notice apples as part of fresh salads or lemon juice as an ingredient in salad dressings.

Benefits of Carrot Combinations

Carrot juices are energy drinks. They provide you with caloric power for that get up and go. Because they are stimulating, they are good to have in the morning or daytime. Depending on the combinations, they can have many specific physiological benefits. Beet juice, for example, is a wonderful stimulant for the liver and parsley is a blood purifier. Sweet potato is an alkalinizer of the bloodstream and a mineralizer that also contains an enzyme for diabetics. Cabbage is a wonderful juice for the stomach that is soothing for ulcers and gas. Cucumbers stimulate the kidneys and parsley is a diuretic. Watermelon's high alkaline fluid content neutralizes acids and flushes toxins out of the kidneys. Spinach stimulates peristalsis. Aloe vera, which is a plant more than a vegetable, is a wonderful detoxifier of the bloodstream and lymphatic system.

Green Juices

Now we leave the land of sweetness and bright colors and enter the serious world of green vegetables. Although some carrot combinations had some greens in them, these juices are all green. Green juices are healing, stabilizing and calming. They give energy by relaxing and centering. If you want a quick pick-me-up, drink carrot juice. But for long-term energy, take a green drink. If you are exhausted, restless or feeling scattered--drink green. Green juice is a quieting drink that is usually taken in the evening. It is perfect for you if you are exhausted. And they can be strong. It is the closest thing to a health cocktail. Imagine how it would change the health of our society if they served these drinks at every corner bar. *"One blood cleanser please, straight up. Hold the cayenne!"*

Green Juice Combinations

Celery Spinach
Celery Spinach Tomato
Celery Spinach Tomato Cabbage
Celery Spinach Tomato Cabbage Dill
Celery Spinach Tomato Cabbage Dill Lemon
Celery Spinach Tomato Cabbage Dill Lemon Garlic
Celery Spinach Tomato Cabbage Dill Lemon Garlic Ginger
Celery Spinach Tomato Cabbage Dill Lemon Garlic Ginger Cayenne
Celery Spinach Tomato Cabbage Dill Lemon Garlic Ginger Cayenne
and Tamari

Wow! This is not just a blood cleanser, it is a body tonifier, nerve tonic, alkalinizer, mineralizer elixir. But if it is not strong enough for you, change the mixture. Add or subtract from the above recipe and do not leave out other important greens such as radish, parsley, green pepper or leafy sprouts such as alfalfa, buckwheat lettuce and sunflower greens. What about the tamari? True it is not a juice. But it is a strained liquid that will not add solids to your system. Here it is added as a flavor enhancer much like a dressing on your liquid salad. The sodium in it helps manage sugar cravings, so if you have too many carrot combos, using green drinks will help balance your blood sugar. If you prefer, substitute tamari with Dr. Bronner's Mineral Broth. This blend of land and sea vegetables from the famous soapmaker, has no added salt and a rich source of vitamins, minerals and flavor. Take it or leave it, the choice, of course, is yours. But try it...you may like it.

How much green juice should you have? A lot fewer than carrot combos or fruit juice. These drinks are indeed like cocktails. You will sip them slowly and 8 to 10 ounces will go a long way. Only one of these will be necessary per day for the average person. If you need strength...go green.

In Respect To The Avocado

We must be thankful for all the avocados in the world and all that they have done to add vitamin A, E, K, essential fatty acids, quality protein and delicious flavor into our lives. But you can't juice it! Just like our friend the banana, this fruit/vegetable yields no water. For some the avocado is the emerald of the fruit kingdom. Hold this gem as your guiding star and look forward to it at the end of your fasting journey.

Home Juicing Remedies

Cold Fighter	Carrot, Lemon, Radish, Ginger, Garlic
Hay Fever Reliever	Carrot, Celery, Radish, Ginger
Immune Booster	Carrot, Celery, Parsley, Garlic
Memory Booster	Carrot, Parsley, Spinach, Kale
Stress Reliever	Carrot, Celery, Kale Parsley Broccoli Tomato
Headache Helper	Carrot, Celery, Parsley, Spinach
Detoxifier	Apple, Beet, Cucumber, Ginger
Antioxidant Cocktail	Carrot, Orange, Green Pepper, Ginger
Anti-Cholesterol	Carrot, Parsley, Spinach, Garlic, Tamari
Liver Cleanser	Carrot, Apple, Beet, Parsley
Gallstones	Lemon (include white pith)
Laxative	Lemon in hot water in first thing in morning
Electrolyte balance	Celery
Liver detox	Wheatgrass
Anti-Inflammatory	Barley Grass Juice powder
Digestive	Pineapple, Papaya
Arthritis	Wheatgrass. All greens.

Chlorophyll—The Healer in Greens

Chlorophyll is the chemical formed by the chloroplast cells of green plants. It is at the beginning of the food chain—the plasma of green plants. Without chlorophyll all animal life on earth would become extinct. Amazingly, this 'blood of plants' is structurally similar to hemin, the protein portion of hemoglobin that carries oxygen. The primary difference is that chlorophyll is bound by an atom of magnesium while hemin is bound by iron. Severely anemic rabbits made a rapid return to normal blood counts once chlorophyll was administered.[1] Somehow the body is able to substitute iron and rebuild the

Chlorophyll
$C_{55}H_{72}MgN_4O_5$

Hemin
$C_{34}H_{32}FeN_4O_4$

blood, in effect giving the anemic patient a transfusion. The chlorophyll in wheatgrass juice elevated blood platelet counts when it was fed to hospitalized patients. [2]

Chlorophyll has long been famous for its ability to heal infected and ulcerated wounds. "Tissue cell activity and its normal regrowth are increased by using chlorophyll."[3] It is an important medicine for healing bleeding gums, canker sores, trench mouth, pyorrhea, gingivitis, even sore throat. Chlorophyll has the unique ability to be absorbed directly through the mucous membranes, especially those of the nose, throat, and digestive tract. It makes a great mouth wash and an excellent dentifrice, especially when used in powder form. Chlorophyll's unique ability to kill anaerobic (odor producing bacteria) is the reason it covers up the smell of garlic, fights bad breath, body odor, and acts as a general antiseptic. These bacteria live without air and are destroyed by chlorophyll's oxygen-producing agents. Dr. Otto Warburg, the 1931 Nobel prize winner for physiology and medicine, concluded that oxygen deprivation, at the cellular level, is a major underlying cause of

GREEN PLANTS –THE SOURCE OF ALL LIFE

Green plants, whether they be wheatgrass or broccoli, get their energy from the sun. Photons of light from sunshine are captured in the cells of green plants called chloroplasts. As the chloroplasts absorb the light, their electrons become excited. They literally dance in the sunshine! The energy they are charged with is stored (like batteries) as ATP (adenosine triphosphate). The ATP then reduces carbon dioxide and water to oxygen and carbohydrates. The oxygen exits the leaf and fills the atmosphere with fresh air. The carbohydrates remain as food. Both the oxygen and carbohydrates become the basic sustenance for all animal life. Were chemists able to duplicate photosynthesis by artificial means, we would have an endless source of power—solar energy.

cancer. At least one alternative cancer therapy today bombards tumors with ozone—highly active oxygen. Unlike many drugs, chlorophyll has never been found to be toxic at any dose.

Chlorophyll may also provide us with protection from low level X-ray radiation from hospital equipment, televisions, computer screens, transmitters and microwaves. No area is totally radiation free. Experiments on guinea pigs in the 1950's demonstrated that radiation-poisoned guinea pigs recovered when chlorophyll-rich vegetables were added to their diet.[4] The U.S. Army repeated this experiment with broccoli and alfalfa and got the same results.[5] But eating green vegetables is not as rich a source of chlorophyll as drinking green juice and the juice highest in chlorophyll is wheatgrass.

What's So Special About Wheatgrass

★ Purifies and Rebuilds Blood   ★ Heals wounds
★ Increases Hemoglobin Production   ★ Is Bacteriostatic
★ Alkalinizes Blood   ★ Detoxifies Cellular Fluids
★ Cleanses the Colon   ★ Heals Intestinal Walls
★ Purges the Liver   ★ Raises Enzyme activity
★ Neutralizes Toxins   ★ Chelates out heavy metals
★ Oxygenates Cells   ★ Elevates 'Chi' or 'Kundalini'

Wheatgrass —The Queen of Juices

Wheatgrass is a popular juice available in juice bars and natural food stores nationwide. Unlike common vegetable juices, it is taken in one ounce doses. To give you an idea of its potency, imagine what it would be like to drink an ounce of garlic juice. Wow! Although it is part of the 9,000 member family that includes the grass on our lawns, wheatgrass and its cousin barley grass, are grown especially for nutritional purposes. These nutritional grasses are some of our finest sources of chlorophyll, but that's only the beginning. Grasses contain many other important pigments, too. There are carotenoids—alpha-carotene and the famous beta-carotene, xanthophylls and zeaxanthin, to name a few. Unfortunately, you can't see them because, just as with beautiful autumn leaves, chlorophyll overpowers the other pigments. There are up to 18,000 units of beta-carotene per ounce of dry grass. This precursor of vitamin A has significant immune enhancing properties including the promotion of T-cells. High levels of this anti-oxidizing nutrient are associated with reduced cancer risk and cardiovascular disease.

Grasses are also abundant in vitamin E and in antioxidants. They have a water soluble form of E called a-tocopherol succinate that has the ability to increase production of prolactin and growth hormone in the pituitary gland.[6] Grasses are rich in vitamin K, the blood clotting vitamin. Grass juice inactivates mutagenic substances found in agricultural chemicals, fertilizers and food additives. [7]

Dr. T. Shibamoto of the University of California, discovered a powerful new antioxidant in barley grass juice called 2"-0-GIV. This new isoflavonoid is both soluble in water and fats and is highly stable. This means it is capable of permeating both the fat and aqueous cell membranes in order to fully protect the cell from the damaging effects of oxidation. According to Shibamoto, 2"-0-GIV is more potent than vitamins E and C, but when taken with them, the effects are profound.[8] Barley grass has all three nutrients in good quantity. Barley grass juice has the potential to prevent arteriosclerosis and is just as effective as the prescription drug Probutol for this disease, without any of the undesirable side effects. [9]

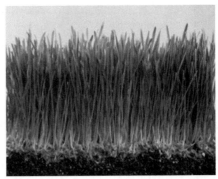

Growing wheatgrass at home is one way to get its highly acclaimed therapeutic benefits.

Barley and wheat grasses are both abundant, inexpensive sources of superoxide dismutase (SOD). This powerful antioxidant and anti-aging enzyme, is a proven anti-inflammatory for arthritis, edema, gout and bursitis. Dr. K. Kubota of the Science University of Tokyo also found two glyco-proteins D1G1 and P4D1 which work alongside SOD but are more heat stable. All three have anti-inflammatory action that is superior to the much touted aspirin. [10]

If fresh grass juice is not locally available, wheat and barley grass juice powders are on the shelves of natural food stores nationwide. Since all research was done with these powders, they stand as a viable nutritive and therapeutic form of the juice. Powdered grass juice products are carefully processed to preserve as many enzymes as possible. Fresh squeezed wheatgrass juice is a veritable enzyme brew of water, oxygen, enzymes, protein, phytochemicals, chlorophyll, carotenoids, fatty acids, trace minerals, all rushing to revitalize you. It is so charged, you can feel it rushing through your body or raising the hair on the back of your neck.

How To Take Wheatgrass

Juicing wheatgrass at home requires a wheatgrass juicer. Only certain juicers can extract the juice from its very woody pulp. These machines range from $300–$600 although manual juicers cost around$100. Volume users drink 3–8 ounces daily and also insert it rectally via enemas and implants[11] for maximum therapeutic effect. However, beginners start with once ounce, and 2 ounces daily are a typical maintenance dose. For volume users, growing your own grass makes the most sense economically. Otherwise, professional growers provide beautifully grown grass to health stores in every major city and you can even have it shipped to your home overnight. Several professional retreat centers offer programs where the grass is grown for you and the juicers are always running *(see Resources)*. Check your local juice bar and health store to see if they sell grass juice by the ounce.

If the intensely sweet taste of grass is too much for you, try mixing it with other green vegetables. Celery is the best match. Its sodium content nicely balances the sugars in young grass. Other favorites are parsley, alfalfa sprouts, spinach, kale, dandelion, and the sprouts of sunflower, buckwheat and pea shoots. Keep it all green. Add some garlic or ginger, too. You'll find it tastes like a liquid salad and the singular taste of grass is gone.

Always drink any kind of grass juice on an empty stomach and wait 30–45 minutes before eating anything solid. Wheatgrass has a strong cleansing effect on the digestive tract. It is practically a green laxative. If you start off taking too much, you could find yourself running to the bathroom. Nausea is common with over-drinking and it is one of the reasons why dosages above 4 ounces are taken rectally. This is somewhat mitigated when mixing it with the celery and the other green juices. Like anything, once you get used to it, you can take more without effect. It's more than the chlorophyll that does this because drinking bottled alfalfa chlorophyll does not cause diarrhea. Fresh wheatgrass is a high frequency enzyme elixir that jumpstarts your system more than other juices. Even superfoods like

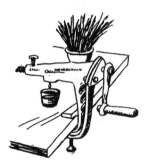

A manual wheatgrass juicer

blue-green algae cannot match the energetic rush or 'chi' of fresh squeezed wheatgrass juice. The secret to drinking wheatgrass juice happily is to gradually increase the dose as you become accustomed to it. Raise your dosage one ounce every few days or every week. Drink only what is comfortable. If you are fighting a serious illness, consider visiting one of the wheatgrass health resorts and following their program.

The Color Of Your Juice (and Food too)

A lot can be said about the individual nutritional characteristics of these wonderful fruit and vegetables, but truly, it is hard to .

remember all the things that they each do. One way to simplify the healing properties of these foods and juices is by designing your drinks, and foods too, around color.

RED FOOD speeds up circulation, creates fire, yang energy (Chinese medicine), heats up your body including hands and feet. Tomatoes, cherries, red cabbage, red peppers, hot peppers, cranberry, watermelon, radish, wheat and rye are some examples.

ORANGE FOOD is anti-spasmodic and is excellent for pains and cramps. It helps strengthen the lungs in polluted environments. Emotionally, it opens up your joy and expansiveness. It promotes vitality and mental clarity. Oranges, carrots, apricots, pumpkin, sesame and pumpkin seeds.

YELLOW FOOD is a motor stimulant, which gets you going faster in the morning. It strengthens nerves, digestion and helps constipation. Lemon, lime pineapple, grapefruit, apple, peach, banana, papaya, mango, yellow squash, corn, butter.

GREEN FOOD is a blood cleanser, bactericide and natural tranquilizer. Nutrifier. All green leafy vegetables and sprouts, wheatgrass, avocado, etc.

BLUE FOOD is for headaches, spiritual, and mental work. It is yin and cooling. Blueberry, plum, grape, potato, celery, parsnip, asparagus, nuts.

How to Extend the Life of Fresh Juice

It's always best to drink your juice right away. Freshly made juice is highly perishable. Any contact with light, heat and air, even at room temperature, commences the process of oxidation. So, it is just a matter of time before your delicious tasting juice turns sour. Realistically, we cannot always make juice whenever we need it. And, if you are drinking juice often, such as on a fast, the process of juicing does indeed become a chore.

Storage is your answer and 'cold' is the key word in storage. You can make enough juice for the whole day or even a couple of days if you can keep it cold enough. The object is to keep the juice as cold as possible without freezing. This means 35 to 38 degrees F. Use a dark, sterile glass bottle that has been pre-chilled. Fill your juice right up to the top so as to reduce the presence of air and oxidation. If you keep your jar sealed, it will stay for about three days. Once you start opening and closing the jar, pouring from it and replacing it in the refrigerator, the contact with air, light and heat commences oxidation, which continues, albeit at a slower rate, even in the refrigerator. The more you open and close the jar, the faster the juice will deteriorate.

The best method of storage for travel is a thermos. Thermoses are designed to retain heat or cold. So begin by pre-chilling your thermos. Then add juice that is also chilled to 35°F. The thermos will maintain this approximate temperature for at about 24 hours, even outside the refrigerator. Thermoses are very handy for transporting your fasting meals to and from work. Just remember, the more you open and close the thermos, the higher the temperature of the juice inside will climb and the quicker it will spoil. Nevertheless, the transportation and convenience of thermos storage make this a superb method. In fact, the absolute best way to extend the life of your fresh juice is to store your thermos inside your refrigerator.

Not all thermoses are created equal! They may be made of glass or stainless steel. Some have more insulation than others. Shop around or experiment on your own to learn how many hours your juice will last. Let your taste be your test. Bad juice, once it has oxidized, will have a 'bite' or tingle on your tongue. It will taste sour or smell foul. It may even coagulate.

The juicing machine itself also plays a role. Again, not all machines are equal. Better machines are able to extract more live nutrients, enzymes and anti-oxidants which act like preservatives and keep the juice stable and extend its life.

Frozen juice is not as preferable as fresh, nevertheless it is another alternative. The process of freezing and thawing destroys some fragile vitamins, enzymes, and cell factors. However, everything is relative. It is not nearly as destructive as pasteurization, canning or irradiating. Frozen juice still tastes good and it is better than buying bottled juices at the store. It is one level removed from being totally fresh and alive. However, if that juice is your whole dinner, such as on a fast, you must have the best. Fasters count on getting every vitamin. Freeze only if you have more juice than you can drink, or if circumstances deem it the best alternative.

Cleaning Fruits And Vegetables

If you are going to all this trouble to fast and carefully make and preserve your juice, you will want to make sure the vegetables are not harboring pesticides, parasites or bacteria. Unfortunately, this may not be easy. While organic carrots are widely available, organic spinach, celery, beets, cucumbers and fruits are harder to get—not to mention more expensive. By properly washing produce, you can remove some of the agricultural chemicals and virtually all bacteria and parasites, which are present even on organic produce.

The most controversial of the above washing methods is the Clorox bath. Controversial yes, but very effective. Even many nutritionists and naturopathic doctors recommend it. Developed by Dr. Hazel Parcells of Albuquerque, New Mexico, this technique works not only because of Clorox's aggressive oxidation, but also, according to Parcells, because of its electromagnetic properties. In addition to destroying parasites and their eggs, it also increases color and flavor and improves freshness. There are even claims that it can remove radiation and lead. Clorox, it seems, works as a chelating agent, extracting pesticides and pollutants from the produce it contacts. Even pesticide workers use it to clean their equipment. True, it is no friend of the environment and if you were to consume Clorox directly, it

Washing Pests Out of Produce	
Lemon Bath Fill your sink with cold water, add four tablespoons of salt and the juice of a lemon. Soak the fruits and vegetables for ten minutes then rinse under cold water. 1/4 cup of white vinegar can be substituted for lemon.	**HCL Bath** Purchase hydrochloric acid from your druggist and pour one ounce into three quarts of water. This is the equivalent of a 1% solution. Soak fruits and vegetables for five to ten minutes and then rinse.
Clorox Bath Use one teaspoon of Clorox bleach per gallon of water. Let your produce sit in the solution for five to ten minutes, then drain and soak again in fresh water for another five minutes. If there is still a Clorox odor after rinsing, rinse once more and let produce air out before consuming.	**Boiling Bath** This method is suitable for all but the most fragile vegetables. Dip the vegetable into boiling water for only 5-10 seconds. That's all you need to kill germs. Remove with tongs. This is also a great way to remove waxes on fruit and vegetables.

would be considered a poison itself. But it is so volatile that it quickly turns into a gas upon contact with air. So if you decide to use it, rinse your vegetables thoroughly and let them air out. If Clorox is there, you will still smell it. If not, it has escaped into the air, leaving you with pure food.

Sprouting is an alternative organic produce—not just bean sprouting in a jar, but real 'kitchen gardening' in professional sprouters that produce different varieties and pounds per week. Sprouts are 100% organic. You don't need a certificate to prove it because you are the farmer. They grow in abundant quantities which makes them perfect for juicing. Where else can you get large quantities of organic produce for only 25¢/lb? Just grow your own! It's not hard and the different flavors will surprise you. Buckwheat, sunflower, alfalfa, garlic, onion, cabbage, pea shoots, broccoli and radish, to name a few. Use these as substitutes for common vegetables. Juice them together with carrots or other veggies. Sprouting is especially economical and nutritious during a fast, but is a valuable adjunct to your cuisine anytime of year.

Symptoms to Look Out For

Sunlight is essential to life on the planet and to our health. Yet, too much of it can cause cancer. In the same way, juicing is a powerful health tool, but here are a few caveats. Do not gorge yourself on juice just as you would not gorge yourself with food. If you find yourself with a voracious appetite, it may be time to stop the fast or switch to non-sweet juices. Don't be alarmed if your urine or stool darkens from the red pigment in beets or green in wheatgrass. Skin can turn yellow/orange from excessive carrot juice. Reduce dosage or switch to green juices. Watch out for berries and other allergic foods. Allergic foods are also allergic juices. Monitor yourself for allergic reactions like itchy eyes or skin. Wheatgrass is not an allergy producing food like wheat. The grass blades have none of the allergic glutinous properties of the grain. However, if you drink too much too soon, you may experience an excitation of symptoms dues to the accelerated rate of detoxification. Stay on the program, but reduce the dosage and frequency to ameliorate the symptoms. Be careful not to confuse elimination symptoms with allergic symptoms. People tend to eliminate in the same places they have long term problems. Those with a tendency to skin rashes, for example, will likely have an aggravation of their symptoms on an intensive juice therapy program. Patients with low blood sugar (hypoglycemia), diabetes, candida, parasites, or other sugar sensitive conditions should avoid sweet juices just as they avoid sweet foods. Cravings for carrot, orange, watermelon, grape and other sweet juices is often an indication of a sugar sensitive condition. You must balance the rate of detoxification with the rate of elimination. While, not all elimination is through the digestive track, colon hydrotherapy and/or enemas are recommended. Expand the other eliminative avenues such as the lungs with aerobic exercise, kidneys with water, skin through sun, air, bathing and massage. This is not a painless process. Typically, a lifetime of bad diet and lifestyle habits such as stress or smoke has generated these conditions. A certain amount of 'toughing it out' is part of the restorative process.

Notes& References

1. *Chlorophyll and Hemoglobin Regeneration After Hemmorrhage*, by J.H. Hughes and A.L. Latner. Journal of Physiology. Vol.86, #388, 1936 University of Liverpool.

2 . Gary's platelet count rose every day for 7 days from 61,000 to 141,000 and the only thing we did differently was administer wheatgrass. That's phenomenal and it's fully documented on the hospital record. —*Leonard Smith, MD., Cancer Surgeon*

3. *Chlorophyll, Nature's Green Magic*, Dr. Theodore Rudolph.

4. *The Influence of Diet on the Biological Effects Produced by Whole Body Irradiation.* M. Lourou, O. Lartigue, Experientai, 6:25, 1950.

5. *Further Studies on Reduction of X-irradiation of Guinea Pigs by Plant Materials.* Quartermaster Food and Container Institute for the Armed Forces Report. N.R. 12-61. by D.H. Colloway, W.K. Calhoun, & A.H. Munson. 1961.

6. *Isolation of a Vitamin E Analog from a Green Barley Leaf Extract That Stimulates Release of Prolactin and Growth Hormone from Rat Anterior Pituitary Cells in Vitro.* By M. Badamchian, B. Spangelo, Y. Bao, Y. Hagiwara, H. Hagiwara, H. Ueyama, and A. Goldstein. Journal Nutrition and Biochemistry. Vol. 5: 145-150. 1994.

7. *Effect on the Several Food Additives, Agricultural Chemicals and Carcinogen.* By Y. Hagiwara, M.D. Presented to the 98th Annual Assembly of Pharmaceutical Society of Japan, April 5, 1978.

8. *A Novel Antioxidant Isolated from Young Green Barley Leaves*, Agricultural and Food Chemistry. Vo. 40, pp. 1135-1138. July, 1992.

9. *Studies on the Constituents of Green Juice from Young Barley Leaves Effect on Dietary Induced Hypercholesterolemia in Rats.* By Y. Hagiwara, K. Kubota, S. Nonaka, H. Ohtake, Y. Sawada. Journal of the Pharmaceutical Society of Japan, Vol. 105, No. 11. 1985. *Inhibition of Malonaldehyde Formation by Antioxidants from 3 Polyunsaturated Fatty Acits.* By J. Ogata, Y. Hagiwara, H. Hagiwara, T. Shibamoto. JAOCS. Vol. 73, no. 5. 1996

10. *Isolation of Potent Anti-Inflammatory Protein from Barley Leaves*, By K. Kubota, Y. Matsuoka, H. Seki, Faculty of Pharmaceutical Sciences, Science Univ. of Tokyo, Japan. Japanese Journal of Inflammation, Vol. 3, no. 4, 1983.

11. For guidelines on how to take wheatgrass enemas and implants see, *Wheatgrass Nature's Finest Medicine* by Steve Meyerowitz. ISBN#1-878736-72-8. 1999 ppbk. 216 pgs $12.95

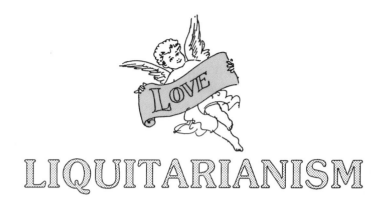

LIQUITARIANISM

In fasting, there are more choices of liquids to consume than just juice or water. Any liquid that is strained, that is without solids, can be taken on a liquitarian fast. This includes herb teas, vegetable broths, nut milks and other clear liquids.

Herb Teas

First of all, let us clarify the term. Herb teas are not true teas at all because "tea" is technically made from the twigs of the tea tree, an evergreen, indigenous to Eastern Asia. Some common twig teas are orange pekoe, java, English tea, jasmine and Ceylon. Herb teas come from green plants and weeds but the term is extended to include tree bark, wood vines and shrubs. They include a wide variety of species that are known for their medicinal and culinary uses. A brew is made of the fresh or dry cut herbs. An accurate description would be to call it an herbal brew. Teas are usually dark in color and contain tannin and caffeine. Tannin is an astringent and an acid and is used to convert animal skins into leather. Tannin is also found in coffee and walnuts. Tea leaves actually contain more caffeine than coffee beans but because more coffee is needed to make a cup, they are ultimately about even in the amount of caffeine per cup. True, herbal brews, however, have no caffeine or tannin and come in many delicious flavors that can be drunk hot or cold. The real function of herb teas is their therapeutic benefits.

Drink your herbal teas as much and as often as you like during your fast. Some teas, like comfrey, are nutritional, meaning they supply vitamins or minerals. Comfrey, for example, supplies calcium. Some are stimulating to the brain or digestive system. Some will help with nausea, bowel movement, gas, appetite, etc. Refer to the herbal tea chart and enjoy your brew.

PROPERTIES OF HERBAL TEAS

EXPELS GAS
Aniseed   Parsley
Caraway   Dill
Fennel   Ginger

PICK ME UP
Peppermint
Spearmint
Basil

APPETITE SUPPRESSANT
Thyme
Fennel
Wheatgrass

STIMULATES DIGESTION
Cinnamon
Cloves
Nutmeg

STIMULATES BOWELS
Cascara Sagrada
Licorice

THIAMINE
Fenugreek
Garlic
Parsley
Catnip
Kelp
Dulse
Raspberry leaves

RIBOFLAVIN
Capsicum
Fenugreek
Parsley
Garlic
Kelp
Dulse

NIACIN
Alfalfa
Burdock
Fenugreek
Parsley
Capsicum
Garlic
Dulse

VITAMIN C
Comfrey
Fennel
Rose Hips
Oregano
Coltsfoot
Elder Berries
Strawberry leaves

VITAMIN A
Fenugreek
Comfrey
Capsicum
Dandelion
Catnip

VITAMIN B-12
Alfalfa
Kelp
Dulse
Comfrey

CALCIUM
Coltsfoot
Dandelion
Horsetail
Nettle
Fennel
Chamomile
Kelp

POTASSIUM
Kelp
Coltsfoot
Comfrey
Peppermint
Yarrow
Garlic
Chamomile

MAGNESIUM
Mullein
Dandelion
Kelp
Peppermint
Parsley
Garlic

IRON
Parsley   Nettle   Strawberry leaf
Fennel   Mullein   Burdock Root   Garlic

Ginger and sage induce perspiration, which has the effect of throwing off toxins and lowering fever. Use in a bath or tea. Ginger and honey is a delicious tea for a variety of stomach complaints. Ginseng is a general tonic that strengthens and gives tone to the stomach, promotes appetite and keeps heat in the body. Vinegar stimulates hydrochloric acid. Honey and vinegar balances the pH of the bloodstream. Licorice is a mild laxative. Cascara Sagrada is a laxative and tonifier for the bowel and stimulant for the liver. Lemon and honey is a liver cleanser and a gall bladder flush. Horehound is good for a sore throat. Cayenne stimulates circulation. Hot apple cider with cinnamon sticks and nutmeg is a delicious way to stimulate digestion. Garlic is a blood purifier and helps fight infections. Barley water stops diarrhea as does bayberry tea, comfrey, yarrow and sassafras. Chamomile quiets the nerves and calms the stomach.

Herbs do many more things than this the extent of which cannot be explored here. Refer to an herb book to learn more about the teas you are drinking. Herbs can be a healthy and refreshing beverage on a fast.

Some other drinks that are not necessarily herbal are the waters made from grains. Rice soaked in water for 24 hours releases its mineral and vitamin content to the water. Use three tablespoons of grain per quart. Be sure to strain before drinking. Barley, wheat and millet are also excellent grain beverages. A drink known as rejuvelac is made from soft wheat berries, which are soaked for three days or until the berries ferment. The fermentation adds friendly bacteria and enzymes to the "brew." Sprout the soft wheat first to make it even more nutritious and again, strain. Another type of grain beverage is made from roasted barley with chicory and is known as herbal coffee. A coffee substitute may be all right to have on your fast depending on its ingredients.

Vegetable Broths

Remember all that delicious water that was left in the pot from boiling vegetables? Do not throw out the water. Give it to a faster. Powdered vegetable broths can be obtained from health stores that make instant broth. Read the ingredients. They should be powdered vegetables, soy protein and sometimes yeast. Some popular brand names to shop for are Arcadia and Vogue. Just heat and enjoy but do not forget to strain out the sediment. If you prefer homemade, gather together potatoes, carrots, garlic, onion, parsnip, parsley, carrot tops, celery, scallions, herbs, miso, seaweeds like kelp and dulse and cook in a big pot with plenty of water. Give the soup to your family and save and savor the broth yourself. By the way, a quick home-cooked broth can be made with a teaspoon of miso paste, ½ teaspoon onion powder, pinch of garlic and cayenne pepper. Add the cayenne after cooking and strain before taking.

Nut Milks

If you are desiring food early on in your fast and are having trouble with your hunger, or if you are on a long term--over 30 days--liquitarian regime, nut milks are for you. These high protein drinks are rich and perfect for when cravings or protein needs exist. They should not be used regularly on short fasts because they are too concentrated and may increase the desire for solid food. But again, they are perfect in the beginning for settling into your fast, on long fasts to carry you through and for coming out of a fast. Milks can be made from almonds, sunflower seeds and sesame. Just blend 1 cup of seeds with 3½ cups of water. Add a teaspoon of honey or maple syrup if you like. Or, use only one cup of water and 2½ cups of apple juice. Like everything else, these milks must be well strained and in this case, will produce a sizable portion of nut meal. Save the meal in the freezer or serve it to your family in salads or desserts. Coconut milk, by the way, is the sweet water that is contained in the coconut shell. It is delicious and nutritious and by all means enjoy it. One caution: Do not make a milk from cashews. Cashews do not have the same kind of fiber and will not strain out. A blend of cashew with water will produce cashew puree containing all the solids and will be a breach of your fast if you drink it.

These nut milks are high in protein, high in fat, are very nourishing and should be used judiciously. High protein drinks on a fast slow down detoxification. Use them only if you need to add calories and nourishment during times of difficulty. Do not confuse these milks with dairy products. No dairy products should be taken on a liquitarian regime. Skim, kefir, clabbered milk halt the detoxification process.

Other Protein Drinks

Again, if you need protein from time to time, there are other drinks you can have in addition to or instead of nut milk. These are superfoods, which are highly dense, rich nutritional sources. They are not manmade or concocted but natural foods taken from plants and other living things. Two such foods are Spirulina and Chlorella. These foods are micro-algae grown in lakes and are the two highest known foods in protein and vitamin B-12. Spirulina is 69 percent protein and contains two and a half times the B-12 of liver. Chlorella has more chlorophyll than any other food grown on land or sea and is a powerful blood purifier. These fresh micro sea vegetables are carefully dried and are taken as powder or tablets. A tablespoon of the powder can be mixed with apple or carrot juice and dissolves readily. No straining is necessary. Some people choose to fast on these foods alone. Both foods suppress appetite.

Nutritional yeast is a product of micro-organisms just like beer, wine and yeasted bread. It is a wonderful source of all minerals, trace elements, RNA, DNA, B vitamins and is 50 percent protein. Some people are allergic to yeast. Avoid this food if you are. Nutritional yeast dissolves readily in juice and does not have to be strained. Again, use in apple or carrot juice.

Soymilk is another possibility for you if you require a rich drink. Soymilk is made by boiling soybeans and pouring off the water. It is not unlike rice water, except that it is commercially made. There are many brands out there and several are pasteurized and homogenized to give it the texture of real milk. This kind is not for you. Just like bottled juices, they are dead foods and, in this case, hard to digest. Fresh soymilk is very healthful, although for some, it is still hard to digest. Only drink soy milk if it suits you.

Rice milk, manufactured by *Rice Dream* is a non-soy alternative. It may be easier to digest than soy, but it is still a complex food and should be tested and or drunk only when diluted. Commercial almond milk is now available and is quite light. None of these drinks are "live foods." Use them occasionally and with discretion.

The Protein Myth

Of all the hundreds of vital health factors, protein has the best press. It is a celebrity among nutrients and the first thing you will be questioned about if you are a vegetarian or on a fast. The real stars of health are oxygen and water.

You can live without dietary protein intake for extended periods, but not air and water. How necessary is protein? Your body uses it in its daily tasks of manufacturing tissues and cells. This is the building phase of metabolism known as anabolism. During a fast, the body's metabolism changes gears and increases the breaking down and cleaning out work—catabolism. Protein is not required for your body's cleansing phase, and as long as you are detoxifying, protein in the usual large quantities will not be needed. Think of building a house vs. cleaning a house. Protein is like wood—essential building material, but not necessary when cleaning.

Protein is in every plant and animal. Even carrot juice has protein. Of course, some foods have more protein than others. But it is a mistake to assume that protein-rich foods are your only sources of protein. True, some of our liquitarian recipe recommendations such as adding a tablespoon of wheatgrass powder or spirulina to your juices or drinking almond milk are increasing your protein intake during your fast, but these are only to be used sparingly. Fasting is a cycle of cleansing and stabilizing and resting. Maintaining balance—alternating cleansing, resting and normal activity—is part of the art of fasting. These liquitarian recipes, with their extra protein, help during times of activity and enable you to stay on your fast longer. The benefits of longer fasting are worth it. Water fasters cannot fast as long and cannot maintain a normal lifestyle. But the fasting process is generally a time to avoid extra protein intake because it slows down detoxification.

A recurring desire for protein, however, indicates that the body is ready to terminate the fast. The cycles of cleansing and stabilizing and cleansing again have turned enough times and your body is wanting to build again. You can never predetermine the exact length of your fast. You must listen to your body and accommodate its needs. The great call of hunger has returned and protein intake should start to increase. But don't get obsessed about protein during your fast. Typically, you need it a little bit on the way into a fast and on the way out, but not much in-between. Listen to your body and not to the fears of your friends.

Apple Cider Vinegar & Other Drinks

Hippocrates, the 'father of medicine,' used natural apple cider vinegar in 400B.C. The early Greeks and Romans kept vinegar vessels to help fight off disease. Even Christopher Columbus brought barrels of vinegar on his voyage to America to prevent scurvy and fight germs. The modern version of this powerful natural antibiotic and antiseptic drink has been distilled, refined, filtered, pasteurized and altogether stripped of its health-giving properties. Use only raw, unfiltered, cloudy vinegar made from organic apples. It should be golden in color and have visible cobwebs of bacterial cultures resulting from the natural fermentation process. The friendly bacteria and natural acidity of this healthy drink act as a powerful intestinal cleanser in addition to helping maintain the body's crucial acid-alkaline balance. While lemon juice also helps balance pH, it doesn't have the friendly bacteria to fight germs and line the intestines. A diet with 2-3 apple cider vinegar drinks daily is famous for dissolving acid crystal buildup in tissues and joints that cause the stiffness of old age and often precipitates out as aching muscles and joints and arthritis. Vinegar is also a superb source of quality potassium. If you like it, you can fast for a few days with vinegar as your primary drink. Shake your vinegar bottle well and add approximately 2 tablespoons to a glass of water. Adjust dosage to your taste. Drink on an empty stomach in the morning and evening or every few hours.

Another acid drink is ascorbic acid—vitamin C powder. Just dissolve it in water and drink up. Vitamin C has various roles in the immune system in addition to the basics—healing wounds and mending bones. An ascorbate form of this vitamin uses minerals such as calcium, magnesium and zinc as carriers for the vitamin.

The drink has a fizzle to it, like Alka-Seltzer, but is pure vitamin C. Add a squeeze of lemon or lime to it and make your own soft drink--au naturel.

Colon Cleansers

Colon cleansers are popular drinks that create a bulk fluid that sweeps through the entire intestinal tract pushing out food from blocked areas on its way. The bulk expands as it goes along and fills up pockets and crevices taking with it old food materials, very much like an intestinal broom. Psyllium seed is the most popular bulking material. It absorbs and expands 10 to 15 times its weight in water. Other similar bulking seeds are flax and chia. They are all part of the gelatinous seed family and literally form a thick gel when wet. These seeds or the powder from them are usually mixed with juice and followed by another full glass or two of juice or water. This is important, because if insufficient water is taken, the gel created by the mixture of seeds and liquid will harden and become very difficult to pass through the intestines.

In drugstores, this type of drink is popularly known by the brand name "Metamucil" among others, and is described as natural-fiber laxative. The fiber here is a soft fiber and very different from bran. The problem with drugstore brands is that they always include sugar. The health store version does not.

There are two forms of psyllium seed--the husks and the meat. The husks are like bran and are coarse. The meat is the meal made from the husked seed and is more gentle and easier to take. Both are non-irritating. The meat, however, surrounds any food that is taken with it and renders it impermeable by the digestive fluids. So do not take anything nutritionally valuable along with your psyllium drink. Take your drinks in the morning before meals or at night at least one and a half hours before bedtime.

The drink is useful on a fast because it acts as an internal colonic. It sweeps through the entire intestinal tract cleaning it as it goes. To make a psyllium colon cleanser, take one rounded teaspoon of powdered psyllium seed and mix it in a glass of juice. Do not use fresh made fruit or vegetable juice for this purpose. The nutrition from these live drinks will become trapped in the mucilage anyway and unavailable for your nourishment. This is one instance where it is preferable to use bottled juice! Blend the drink in the blender and add a banana for flavor. While fasting, you can take as many as three to six drinks per day. Start with one and increase only when and if it feels comfortable. This drink is very, very filling and will cause distension of the abdomen, so do not be alarmed. It is just a lot of healthy fiber. If you are a beginner, it may make your fasting easier by giving you a feeling of fullness in your stomach.

Psyllium seed can be expensive and it is not everybody's favorite tasting drink. If you prefer, you can make a less expensive, good tasting drink on your own with chia and flaxseed. Blend one tablespoon of chia and one tablespoon of flax with 2 cups of apple juice and one half banana. Blend thoroughly. If the drink is too thick, add more water or juice. This drink has the advantage of using both the husk and the meat of the seed, tastes better than psyllium, and costs less, too.

Whichever drink you choose, stay on the regimen for 3 to 6 days before stopping, break for 2 or 3 days, then repeat. You will find your movements are long and full and the elimination is quite thorough. Some preparations add different herbs to the mixture or bentonite, a clay. These help draw poisons from the intestines or stimulate peristalsis.

When to Use Vitamins and Herbs

Of course our fast, even our liquitarian fast, maintains that no matter what we drink, there be no solid food. This, right from the start, limits us to supplements that completely dissolve and excludes gelatin capsules. But before we start taking vitamin C and other vitamins that go into solution, we must determine the type of fast we are on and the goals that we have.

Basically, a fast is for the quieting of the whole digestive tract and the balancing of our natural chemistry without the influence from foods, etc. When we start taking vitamins, we disturb that natural balance. If your purpose, however, is to detoxify or to work on a particular health problem, you may choose to add certain herbs or vitamins that accelerate these processes. That would assist your fast, not interfere with it. For, in this instance, your goal is healing, not fasting. Fasting is the means to achieve your goal and if you must bend the rules slightly to get better results, then these minor infringements are acceptable. This would permit, for example, the addition of powdered herbs such as echinacia or golden seal to your green vegetable juice to increase the healing powers of the juice and support the immune system.

What vitamins are appropriate to take? Only the water soluble vitamins are acceptable on a fast and preferably only vitamin C. If you need to take a specific B vitamin for a particular health problem, for example B-1, then do it under supervision. In this case, the vitamin is being used therapeutically as a drug. But if you just want to take a shot-gun vitamin--a pill that includes all the B-vitamins in one tablet--please don't. You do not need supplements during a fast. Your fresh juices supply you with all that you need. Vitamin C is the only exception because of its influential role in detoxification and immune system support. But, in general, you do not need vitamin and mineral supplementa-tion. In fact, supplements can unbalance the delicate chemistry in your system.

One more thing--avoid aspirin and Tylenol (acetaminophen) on a fast. These drugs quash symptoms, but they do not cure anything and interfere with the natural body chemistry. Gout, arthritis, arteriosclerosis are chronic conditions that may not have developed if toxic crises were allowed to run their course unimpeded by drugs. Take enemas, baths, use heating pads on your head, rest or go to sleep, but avoid these medicines. Of course, all medicines and drugs are eschewed on a fast. One couple this author counseled, was fasting but smoking marijuana. The effect of this and other drugs is increased in a system where no other external nutriments are being taken. It stresses the liver, which has to detoxify the nicotine and THC and slows down the whole detoxification process.

Cold Drinks vs. Hot Drinks

During your fast, one of the decisions you will face is what to drink. Should you have water, carrot juice, a fruit juice, a green cocktail, an herbal tea, a hot broth...? One of the factors that will help you decide is whether you want your drink to be hot or cold. This narrows the field. But if you choose cold, you must avoid using ice cubes or drink-ing iced drinks. These are not healthful at any time of year, but during fasting when your stomach is contracted and relatively dormant, the addition of iced liquids is a shock to the system that it is ill-prepared to handle. Avoid ice cubes. If you are hot, go for a swim instead. The same is true for hot drinks. Very hot drinks can be irritating, especially to a sleeping stomach. Hot is okay, but not too hot. Hot coffee, just in case you were wondering, is not on the list of liquitarian beverages. Neither is iced coffee or a cold beer.

Don't Forget Water!

Please don't. Just because a liquitarian has so many wonderful choices does not mean that he/she should exclude the number one fasting drink--water. Water is a superb solvent and a flushing agent and cleanser for all the other liquids that are working your kidneys, bladder and digestive tract. Water also contains natural electrolytes, which are acids, bases and salts that conduct our bio-electricity through our nervous system. Don't forget that water is very nourishing providing vital minerals and trace minerals. Water is healthful...that is, of course, as long as it is pure water.

Quality of Water

One of the most important issues of fasting is the quality and type of water consumed. It is often overlooked because of the popular belief that water is water. It isn't!

Water must be pure. We cannot go through the trouble and effort to cleanse our bodies and simultaneously proceed to pollute it with tainted H_2O. Pollution is a big problem but one to which many people close their minds because they do not have the answers. This behavior prefers to deny the issue rather than take on the formidable effort of resolving it. But water pollution is clearly a national, indeed global, problem. You may purchase water in gallon jugs, make your own with a distilling machine, or filter it. Within these choices come other questions. Is bottled water safe to drink? Will the filter remove everything? Doesn't the distiller make dead water?

True, distilled water is lifeless. First of all, it is made by boiling water, which destroys bacteria through sterilization. Bottled water, however, may not be what it is purported to be. Misleading advertising and bogus brands have given the industry a damaged name. *Purified* water passes the water through a very sophisticated carbon block. The block itself is so dense that even bacteria cannot crawl through.

One of the most controversial topics in the health field today is the dispute over whether to drink distilled, spring, or filtered water. It is partly a question of what is natural. Spring water is of course natural, but is it pure? In today's polluted environment and competitive commercial world, how can we be certain that we are truly getting what the label tells us. True, filtered water leaves the healthful minerals in, but, for the most part, it cannot remove fluorides, nitrates, sulfates or sodium. If the latter are not an issue in your area, then high density, carbon block filters are a suitable choice. A few carbon block filter manufacturers have added media which can remove fluorides and nitrates. Distilled water, however, is the primary choice for removing these "ions," but it also removes everything making the water, "dead". Dead water means it is sterile containing no life forms. Reverse osmosis is a relatively new technology that removes salts, fluorides, nitrates as well as the common organic pollutants. Water is passed through membrane which slowly filters out the pollutants. Unfortunately, the membrane is subject to the hardness/softness of water, acidity/alkalinity, turbidity and thus is unable to give consistent purification in all locations and the performance life of the membrane is not entirely predictable.

Should you be drinking dead water on your fast? Probably not. If your water does not provide nutrients, it is not going to feed you on a water fast, since water is your only source of nutrients. Nevertheless, distilled water helps to cleanse your kidneys, bladder and bloodstream and is a natural chelator. If you are taking juices, then you probably do not have to worry about the minerals you are not getting because water is not your only mineral source. In fact, a glass of carrot juice will supply you with more calcium then 50 glasses of spring water. Any of the waters then would be suitable on a juice fast as long as they were pure. Spring water, on the other hand, or any pure water with minerals, would be mandatory on a water fast, since this is your only source of minerals. Water with minerals could come from your own carbon block filtered water or from reconstituted distilled water. What is reconstituted distilled water? It is distilled (sterile) water that has been remineralized. This can be done by adding 3 grains of rice to one gallon of distilled water. The grains release their minerals, vitamins and enzymes in the water making it alive. Other possible methods are to leave the distilled water in the sun to charge and energize it--and you, too.

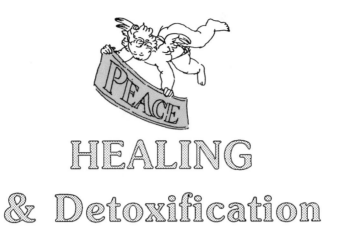

HEALING

& Detoxification

The Cycle of Healing and Detoxification

When you fast, you are on nature's operating table. The body changes hats. Instead of being in the business of receiving, processing, storing, analyzing, assimilating, discriminating and discarding, it shifts to the job of house cleaning, removal, sanitizing, refurbishing and renewal. It is a big job and it is not without its inconveniences especially when there is someone living in the house.

No one ever said that fasting was 100% easy. It is probably easier than you think. Actually, fasting is very easy, it is just healing that is hard! In fact, healing can make you sick. Take a look at the following symptoms:

SYMPTOMS OF A HEALING EVENT

Rash	*Headache*
Eczema	*Faintness*
Acne	*Fever*
Nausea	*Diarrhea*
Weakness	*Muscle Aches*
Dizziness	*Bad Breath*
Hot Flashes	*Stuffed Nose*
Fatigue	*Running Nose*
Bronchitis	*Irregular Heartbeat*
Asthma	*Irregular Menstruation*

Oy! Is this a fast or a flu? Actually, symptoms during a healing event on a fast can be just like those of a flu. Poisons make you sick twice--on their way into the body and on their way out. The liver has been a real pal to store them for you all these years, but the spring cleaning, called fasting, has exposed the cobwebs. The colon has happily held decades worth of polluted material, but when you start opening up those dark and dingy corners, they unfold all their muck and mire. How do you get poisons out of the body? First, they have to get back into circulation again since they have been immobilized for years. Once in circulation, they go around for a while looking for the way out. They may travel through the head (ouch! what a headache). They may try to get out the skin (rashes, acne, boils, sores, eczema). They may attempt a trip down the bowel (diarrhea). They may try to escape through the lungs (bronchitis, asthma), or the kidneys (pain on urination, bad odor). What if they cannot escape so easily? The longer they stay around, the weaker and more fatigued you feel. Fevers are very common. Anything you can do to speed up the house cleaning will be to your benefit. (See *Methods of Detoxification* p. 77.)

These periods of great discomfort are called healing events and come and go on a regular cycle during a long fast. They are also referred to as healing crises since they represent a climax of detoxification and a catharsis or cleaning event. They may arrive as often as every 10 to 14 days. For your peace of mind, know that healing events are relatively short. They generally last one to three days, although they can run longer. You may feel very sick, but the time in between each event is pure energy--you feel great. The more you assist elimination, the quicker these "sick" days will pass and the milder their symptoms. When you are experiencing a healing crisis keep in mind, the greater the release, the greater the healing and the greater the gain. The area of congestion in your body determines the type of eliminative crises.

Caution must prevail. If your symptoms are too severe and frequent, if your fever is too high, if you do not have confidence in what you are doing or proper professional guidance, then, and only then, should you consider breaking your fast. Breaking the fast will dilute the poisons in your bloodstream with food. It will relieve the stress on your system. The crisis is temporarily over. But you have not resolved the problem of what to do about the poisons that made you so sick. They remain inside you, just suppressed. Juice fasting generally creates milder healing events than water fasting. Drink plenty of fluids and use all the methods of detoxification (next chapter) available to dilute the poisons. Lie down and wait for it to pass. Sweat it out. Rest, sleep, rest. Do not stand up to quickly else you will get dizzy. Try not to be alarmed. In general, fasting is more joyous than uncomfortable and healing events are often followed by periods of euphoria.

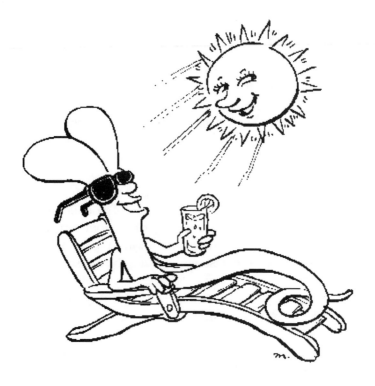

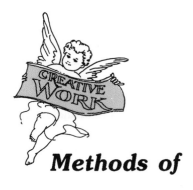

Methods of

DETOXIFICATION

The Organs Of Elimination

Help your organs and they will help you! As mentioned, there are several ways in which toxins can get out of the body. You can help by making sure the path is clear and by using your royal influence to speed things along. Who told you that fasting was just the abstinence from food? You can't get off the hook without some hard work! Let us take each of the organs, discuss their eliminative functions and see what you can do to help.

Lungs

Oh, for a breath of fresh air! Yes, just breathing will help your lungs. Though you may not realize or want to know it, your lungs take in pounds of pollutants and are constantly eliminating volumes of toxic gases each minute. Remember, oxygen is our most important nutrient. It is the front line between life and death. You can fast and do without food.

You can even do without water for a while, but you cannot do without air. Pay respect to your lungs and they will breath life into you.

First of all, let's build those muscles. Although you may not think of it, your lungs are made of muscle tissue and should be exercised! One of the best ways to exercise your lungs is to take up the tuba. If the tuba is bigger than you, try the coronet. If you are not musical, try a balloon or a rubber raft. That's right, go blow! If that is too rigorous, just breath deeply. We use only one third of our lung capacity for most of our daily activities. How can we reach the other two-thirds? Breathe deeply.

Some of the best exercises for breathing can be found in the science and practice of Yoga. Yoga is more an "innercise" than exercise. With only ten or fifteen minutes of yoga breathing per day, you can distinctly influence your detoxification and overall health. First, just breathe in and out in three stages filling up the top, middle and bottom lungs. Go slowly and rest briefly at either end. Or, you may force air out of your lungs in sharp diaphragmatic breaths known as *Kapalabhati* or sharp in and out bellow breaths known as Bhastrika. Or, you may close one nostril with your finger and breath through the other and keep breathing while alternating nostrils. Consult your yoga teacher or yoga book for complete guidance on these powerful exercises.

If you want to let off some steam, do it with a vaporizer. Vaporizers add warm moist air to your environment, which softens waste materials and affords easier breathing. Add eucalyptus, tea tree oil, menthol or specific herbs like comfrey to help with the elimination. Vaporizers are built to house any concoction you want to send into your lungs.

They are different from humidifiers. Humidifiers usually send cold moist air into the general room. Most do not take medicines (it clogs the machine). However, it is important to have properly humidified air, especially in the Winter when home heating systems dry out indoor air. Ultrasonic humidifiers use sound waves to break up water droplets into a fine mist. They do not develop mold and mildew inside like the traditional belt humidifies. You may be allergic or sensitive to mold. But ultrasonic machines are controversial because of the white mineral (calcium) dust they deposit in the house from the atomization of water. They also use sound waves which is a questionable area in terms of their effect on human health. Humidifiers that use a heating element to vaporize the air, are the preferred "low-tech" alternative. Dehumidifiers, by the way, are also very healthful because they remove mold and mildew in a house by removing the moisture on which they thrive. They are especially useful in old wood houses in rural areas and in summertime when humidity is high.

You can also help your lungs by drinking teas. Fenugreek, comfrey, lobelia, pleurisy root, elecampane and horehound are just a few of the teas you can use. Refer to your herb guide or herbal teacher for complete instructions. And do not forget to exercise. Mild aerobic exercises, those that excite the breathing, are one of the best ways to detoxify the lungs. (See *Exercises*, p.86)

Skin

The skin is our largest eliminative organ. Every pore of your body is an opening, an escape route for waste material. Don't ignore your skin. Brush it, aerate it, scrub it and bathe it. If your skin feels good, so do you. There are two ways you can use your skin to expel wastes: internal stimulation and external stimulation.

External stimulation is the washing and brushing we mentioned. Natural fiber brushes rubbed on the skin leave it rosy and tingling clean. Circulation comes alive and carries away poisons looking for an escape route. By raising the circulation to the skin, you provide an outlet for toxins. Loofas, a natural sea-fiber brush, are also excellent.

Give your skin air. Avoid synthetic clothing because it can prevent proper ventilation and irritate the skin especially if you are sensitive. Natural cottons breathe best and are non-allergenic. Caveat Emptor. Some synthetics described as non-allergenic are not at all. Be careful. Whenever you can, wear as few clothes as possible. Go outside and expose your skin to the sun and air. This is not a recommendation to get a sunburn, just to air out your body.

Internal stimulation involves doing things that stimulate elimination through the skin without actually doing anything to the skin directly. Saunas and steam baths are an example. Steam baths are preferred on a fast because the hot dry heat of saunas is very enervating. If you can only do a sauna, limit yourself to the minimum you can tolerate. A steam bath, also called a Russian bath, however, adds moisture to your lungs and your whole body. It softens the skin and the heat stimulates circulation throughout. Your pores excrete sweat and toxins flow out along with it. Take a brief cold bath for further stimulation, then back to the steam.

At home, just take a hot bath. Do not make it too hot if you are in a weakened condition. Use Epsom salts or dead sea salts, herbs like ginger, cayenne and sage or equivalent products. These baths make you sweat and can help in mitigating a headache, fever, skin problems, etc. Salty water creates an osmotic flow from the fluids of your lymphatic and circulatory systems to the bath water. If you use Epsom salt, do not be afraid to throw the whole 4 pound container in the tub. Some people add baking soda to increase the cleansing action on the skin. Epsom salt is also a muscle relaxant and after 10 to 20 minutes, (spend only as long as you can tolerate), get out and quickly run under the covers and sweat, sweat, sweat. Do this once a day or as much as possible. Mineral baths at certain health spas are also healing in a similar way. Take advantage of them. All these baths help moderate the discomfort of your healing events.

If you are near an ocean, don't hesitate to go in, cold or not. Ocean water is salty and a wonderful cleanser. Your skin will tingle and feel squeaky clean. Lie in the sun afterwards. If your skin gets too dry from sun and salt, rub yourself down with vitamin E oil or aloe vera gel. This is not a sunscreen, just a healing lubricant.

Kidney

The kidneys have the primary role in eliminating fluid wastes from the body and continuously purify the bloodstream. These two organs, at the small of the back, rarely get a rest, even on a fast, unless it is a fast of distilled water. Because distilled water has no mineral or nutritional content, it acts as a flush for the kidneys. Instead of the kidneys working to purify the water, the water purifies the kidneys. However, in comparison to food and drink, any water is a relief to the kidneys.

Many herbs are specific to the kidneys because of their ability to cleanse, increase the flow of urine (diuretics) and even dissolve kidney and bladder stones. Some of these are juniper berries, parsley, wild carrot, gravel root and uva ursi. Juices are extremely effective. Use watermelon rind, parsley, cranberry, cucumber, celery, aloe vera, wheatgrass, dandelion, strawberry and asparagus. Avoid cooked oxalic acid vegetables such as spinach, rhubarb and swiss chard which can build up oxalic acid crystals in the body, often depositing them in the kidneys and bladder.

Hot and cold compresses on the kidneys help relieve aches. Vitamin C is acknowledged even by orthodox medicine as an aid in kidney and bladder infections. Asthma is often related to kidney dysfunction. Asthma sufferers, give your kidneys some sun. Warm sunshine is very healing and it is not just the heat of the sun that helps your kidneys but also the chromatherapy. Let the sun play its melody of healing rays on your back. Fast. Drink distilled water. Give the kids a rest!

Liver

The liver is probably the most important detoxifier of all the organs because it takes poisons, neutralizes them, and what it cannot render harmless, it stores. The essential result is the same because it protects us from harm. However, too much bad diet for too long is more than our livers can handle, and you will see the symptoms of these excesses in the quality of your skin and hair. When fasting, the liver gets very busy. It fields and filters poisons coming to it from other parts of the body while at the same time releasing its own unwanted toxins. Thankfully, it is temporarily off the hook from processing new food. Release the liver from its heavy burden. Fast, cleanse and purge it with raw juices, herbs, exercises and manipulation. Let the liver live!

Juices for the liver are wheatgrass, carrot, beet, dandelion, parsley, lemon, grapefruit, apple and spinach. A teaspoon of olive oil added to lemon or grapefruit juice stimulates the release of bile by the gall bladder. (The gall bladder is joined to the liver.) Herbs can be used effectively for the liver in teas and in hot and cold compresses placed over the area. Some of these are golden seal, mandrake, cascara sagrada, black cohosh, and bitterroot to name a few. Consult your herb book or herbologist for proper use. Place a moist heating pad on the liver to stimulate circulation and detoxification. Or shine a red light on it to stimulate it, lemon to loosen and cleanse it, and green finally to relax and heal it. Sunshine and exercise are excellent for your liver.

Visit your masseuse. A liver and an intestinal massage, as well as a full body massage, is one of the best things you can do on your fast. The liver provides us with a real advantage over the other major organs because we can reach it. Physical manipulation of the liver is one of the best ways to assist detoxification because it mechanically stimulates the organ, in addition to the help of juices and herbs that chemically stimulate it. A good masseur/masseuse can knead and pump the liver like a baker kneads bread. Be careful not to do too much. You only want to release what you can tolerate. Start your massages slowly and gently. Work closely with your masseur/seuse. Let them know how you are feeling. If used judiciously, a massage every day can more than double the accomplishment of your fast in the same amount of time. Viva la masseuse! Viva la liver.

Colon

The colon eliminates solid wastes and absorbs water from foods. When food first enters the small intestine, it is in a moist semi-solid state. The colon absorbs the moisture from the food leaving solids to be eliminated from the body. Throughout the entire passage of the intestinal tract, peristalsis, the wavelike motion of the intestines, keeps the food moving along to the exit, the anus. When fasting, peristalsis quiets down almost entirely as the intestine empties. This does not mean, however, that there is no more waste. The colon is riddled with pockets (diverticuli), turns and convolutions wherein waste collects. These areas are rarely cleaned because of the regular passage of enormous quantities of food. During fasting, these pockets begin to empty and in addition, toxic fluids being eliminated in other parts of the body, make their way down to the colon. Because of the lack of solid food and peristalsis, these poisons are frequently re-absorbed by the colon instead of eliminated. This process is frequently the cause of headaches, fatigue and skin problems, to name a few. Any way you can assist the elimination from the colon, will be to your advantage.

The most direct and best way to hasten the removal of waste from the colon is through the use of colonics and enemas. These techniques simply involve the use of water as a wash much in the same way a douche cleans the vaginal area. A discussion of the differences between the two and their relative advantages will follow. Psyllium seed drinks and other bulk drinks that gel up in the intestines (See *Colon Cleansers*, p.66.) also work effectively to maintain movement of waste material through the colon.

Herbs can also stimulate peristalsis and nourish the colon. Some herbs like senna, cascara sagrada and mandrake, actually work as irritants which the colon attempts to expel along with other wastes. Herbs like rhubarb root, peppermint, golden seal, aloe and wheatgrass act as a tonic to heal the colon. A tea made from flaxseed is a wonderful laxative as are the raw juices of celery, apple, carrot, rhubarb, spinach, prune, fig, raisins and the lactobacillus cultures.

An intestinal massage does wonders before an enema or colonic. Exercise and deep breathing should also be a part of your total colon health program.

Other Effects

During fasting, your tongue, teeth and gums may develop a coating. If you are on a juice fast, brush your teeth or use mouth wash. If you are on a water fast, use only salt and bicarbonate of soda as a mouth wash and tooth paste. You can scrape your tongue with a spoon or a special tongue scraper available in East Indian supply stores.

Your eyes may develop encrustations especially in the morning or they may tear. Ears may clog up with wax or dirt. Not surprisingly, your nose may drip, run, congest or sneeze. These are all avenues of elimination. Keep normal hygiene practice in these areas, especially during the fast.

If you feel nauseous, lie down and rest. If the sensation refuses to go away and is accompanied by a headache, induce vomiting. Regurgitation may be difficult for some but it is not ugly and in some instances it is the most expedient way to eliminate poisons from the body. One should know how to induce vomiting even as a general health practice in case of emergency such as poisoning. Several glasses of warm salty water helps. Take lobelia tea, a strong herbal emetic (causes vomiting), if necessary. Wash hands, bend over toilet or sink and tickle the back of the throat. Rinse and continue until the majority is eliminated. Vomiting will cause heavy perspiration as part of the eliminative process. Lie down afterwards and sleep or rest. You will feel much relieved. You can get rid of a lot of poisons easily and quickly this way although it is more rigorous and less romantic. Yogi's actually swallow purified cloth and pull it back out as part of a stomach cleansing process called *Dhauti*. (In case you want to rush right out and do this, we recommend consulting a yoga professional or book first.) Regurgitation is not a requirement, but it is sometimes the most expedient way to deal with fever, headache, nausea and general malaise during a healing crisis.

If you have a headache, put your feet in a hot foot bath filled with mustard or cayenne. The bath draws blood away from the head and relieves pressure. Ice packs on the head are also helpful. If sinuses are congested, a sinus (facial) heating pad that surrounds the eyes and nose can be beneficial. The pad should supply moist heat and may ease up the congestion. Sometimes a hot compress to the liver or intestines is also beneficial since headaches are often symptoms that reflex to those organs.

Exercises for Detoxification

Exercise should be an important part of your health program whether fasting or not, but it is particularly important to include during fasting. Aerobic exercises are those that demand significant increases in respiration and are the most important. These include swimming, biking, walking, trampolining and gentle dancing. Yes, running and jogging are also aerobic, but are conspicuously left out because they are too strenuous for a fast. Exercise, after all, demands energy and your fast, as we have discussed requires the conservation of energy, thus the only exercises we should be considering are those that facilitate elimination without creating additional stress. Swimming and walking are two of the finest exercises in that respect. The lungs increase their activity oxygenating cells and expelling gaseous wastes. Trampolining is another fine exercise because it shakes up the lymphatic system, helps remove fluid wastes and does not jar the skeletal system. Running does bang at the ankles and knees and causes stress on the heart muscle. Running and jogging are wonderful exercises with many advantages, but not at this time.

Yoga, while not exactly aerobic, is a wonderful practice during a fast. There are specific yoga positions that stimulate and massage the colon, small intestine, thyroid, liver, kidneys, adrenals and lower back, etc. Whether they make you go upside down or just cause compression and release in a given area, they are mild yet very effective. Yoga can squeeze toxins out of muscles and joints. And do not forget pranayama, the deep breathing exercises that empty the lungs and oxygenate the whole body.

Be careful with exercise. Fasting is not the time to lift weights or do heavy aerobic dancing. You must choose your exercises in the same way you would if you were pregnant. Remember, when fasting, your body is half asleep. Jarring exercises like jogging and jumping rope will shock, stress and enervate more than achieve your goal. Do not forget: the aim of these exercises is not to build strength, but to assist detoxification. Above all, you must avoid exhaustion. Be conscious of exercising to the point of stimulation but not enervation.

The Large Intestine

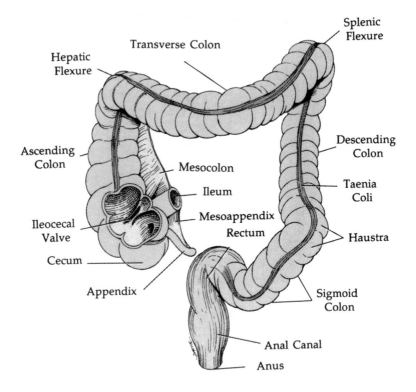

Colonics And Enemas

Yuck!

Let's face it. This is not everybody's most appetizing subject. The mere mention causes faces to cringe. This is unfortunate because it should be just another part of our personal hygiene like cleaning the wax out of our ears or the dirt under our nails. It is no more or less ugly than a vaginal douche. Ultimately, it is too important to our health to carry such a stigma.

Try It, You'll Like It!

It sounds like the punch line of an old commercial, but in this case, it really is true. Although few people go into a colonic session willingly or joyfully, the vast majority walk out ready to do it again. The reason is simple. There is an instant feeling of freshness. You can see and feel the results.

Advantages

Both colonics and enemas simply perform a rinsing of the colon with water. There are dozens of medical techniques that are more invasive and more painful. Nonetheless, people cringe at the thought of enemas because of the psychological inhibitions involved in confronting one's own waste. It is a cultural problem as well. No community wants to have their trash burned in their backyard, so public waste is often shipped miles away. It is becoming a major health and environmental issue that we will have to face as a society. And it all starts with the individual. The fear of enemas and colonics for most people has to do with lack of knowledge about them. Most of us simply do not recognize that, essential to our internal mechanism, is the production of waste. As soon as we accept the responsibility of our own waste management, then the stigma is gone and our health is better for it.

If you want to achieve good health, you cannot go around for life ignoring your bowels--or any other part of your body for that matter. Especially during fasting, it is imperative to keep the bowels clear. As we mentioned earlier, solid waste still comes down the intestines even though you are not eating, but because there is no bulk to help move it along, it often collects and gets reabsorbed leading to headaches, fatigue and other discomfort. This process is known as auto-intoxication. Preventing auto-intoxication and assisting elimination is part of your job during fasting. Regular colon cleansing can speed up detoxification and actually shorten your fast. One colonic can be worth two days of fasting, i.e., it would take two days to remove an equivalent amount of waste through normal body elimination. Why fast for longer than you have to? Speed up detoxification with a colonic or an enema. You will feel better, too.

Difference between Colonic and Enema

You may already be familiar with an enema bag. You can purchase it in every drug store in the personal hygiene section next to douches and hot water bottles. Watch what you buy--there are two kinds--a chemical one and a water one.

The chemical enema is small and has a one time use. The chemicals act as agents to stimulate the evacuation of the bowels. This is for people who cannot move their bowels and equivalent to taking castor oil or other laxatives. This is not recommended and does not suit our purpose. Choose the water bag enema, the two quart size. The enema procedure simply allows the water to enter slowly and exit the colon little by little alleviating solid wastes in the process. You lie down to take the water in and go to the toilet to release. There are no needles or sharp points or chemicals, just water. And the colon is used to water since part of its main job is to remove water from our food.

Having a colonic is a similar procedure although on a grander scale and with the assistance of a professional. It takes place in a therapist's office and is usually performed by a trained individual who may be a nurse, a physical therapist or simply a colonic therapist. Most have their own offices or share offices with masseurs, acupuncturists, chiropractors or naturopaths. Some operate in medical doctors' offices, an indication of the acceptance of this procedure into the mainstream. The advantage of a colonic is that you lie down and relax your body, especially your abdomen, while the therapist controls the entrance and exit of the water. The solid wastes also exit through the tubing so there is no need to get up to go to the toilet. Because it is so efficiently organized, more water is able to be taken in a shorter amount of time. A colonic usually sends about 5 gallons of water in and out of the colon in a typical 45 minute session. Compare that to only 2 quarts in an enema in almost the same amount of time! Obviously, a more thorough job is done in the colonic in terms of sheer volume, but the operator also massages the abdomen, which aids in loosening up impacted material. The extra volume also helps get into the pockets (diverticuli) and folds of the colon and the water penetrates deeper into the intestinal tract. Also, remember that you are laying down and relaxed so your muscles are working with the procedure more than with a home enema. One clarification: the five gallons do not go in all at once. The influx of water is regulated according to your comfort. You participate in the whole process and your therapist is very much in touch with your comfort. Most people who are squeamish about this subject, like colonics even better than enemas. In some ways they are like getting a rubdown. Although there are moments of discomfort, you often feel refreshed and energized afterwards, making the total experience positive.

How And When

One of the advantages of the enema is that you can do it at home according to your own schedule and at no expense. During a fast, enemas should be taken on a regular basis whether that be daily, once every two days or even once every three days. A colonic once or twice a week during a fast is recommended. The more you do it the better you will feel and the easier it gets. Once the bowels are cleared, enemas get quicker and more efficient. Rinse your bag to make sure it is clean, then fill it with lukewarm, purified water. Lubricate the enema tip and anus area with lubricating jelly, available in any drugstore, Crisco or other salve of your preference. Get in position on the toilet and release a small amount of water first to relieve any air pockets. Plant the enema tip fully into the anus and regulate the rate of flow with the small valve. Lie down adjacent to the toilet in any comfortable position you prefer, on your back, stomach, or any side. Initially, the back or left side is preferred. On repeated enemas, after the bowels are clear, you will find alternating positions helps to move the water around and into pockets and folds. When you feel the urge to release, go back to the toilet. During the first enema, you may get up and down a few times before finishing the entire bag. After the first or second enema, you will probably be able to take the entire two quarts in one sitting.

Exotic Enemas

Though you may find it hard to believe, some people become very attached to their colon treatments! Even when not fasting, you can take enemas or colonics periodically as part of your regular detoxification program. A colonic once a month or every six weeks is very helpful. There are many things you can put into the water--herbal brews, wheatgrass, vinegar, acidophilus, polarized water to name a few. The herbs help to stimulate the liver and cleanse or tonify the colon depending on the ones you choose. (Refer to *Herb Teas*, p. 57 or to your herb guidebook.) Wheatgrass also stimulates the liver to purge itself, neutralizes poisons and alkalinizes an acidic colon. Acidophilus powder in the enema water replaces some of the natural friendly bacteria that are flushed out. Vinegar helps maintain proper pH of the colon for those people who do not produce enough hydrochloric acid and whose intestinal tract is too alkaline. Cold water is thought to contract the muscle tissue and stimulate peristalsis. Hot water should never be used because it is too much of a shock to the colon and can result in the reabsorption of pollutants. Warm water will help loosen some solids and is preferred. If you are using herbs, make your enema water only as strong as a cup of light tea. For wheatgrass, add only one or two ounces of juice. For vinegar, use one ounce and use a teaspoon for acidophilus.

Is It Harmful?

The most controversial issue preventing the wider acceptance of enemas and colonics is the accusation they ruin the body's natural ability to eliminate. Overall, this is not the case. Like anything, these treatments can be misused. There are enema fanatics out there who take enemas or colonics all the time, fasting or not. Yes, if you remove the need for muscular action to take place, then those muscles stop working and can eventually weaken. But this is in cases of negligence and misuse. Even in cases of long fasts where enemas may be elected on a daily basis, if you had normal muscular activity before, you will have it again. The sphincter muscle can be exercised simply by voluntary contraction and release. Repeat the movements for one minute two or three times per day. This sets up a signal to start the peristalsis action just like one domino falling starts the movement of all the others. To work on the muscles of the lower abdomen, use a slant board. Lay on the board with your feet higher than your head and lift your legs up or bring your knees to your chest. Do as many motions as you can. The slant board position allows your muscles to exercise while not working against gravity.

Another possible area for a problem is the sigmoid section of the colon, the part just above the rectum. If the lower (descending) colon is congested or the flexure (point where colon turns) is blocked, the water may just fill up the area causing a ballooning of the sigmoid. If this problem reoccurs often enough, it can weaken and stretch the muscles in that area. Extension tubing for enema tips is available through some pharmacies and surgical supply stores. The longer (30 inch) tube passes beyond the sigmoid colon and eliminates the potential for this problem. The extension tube also has the advantage of riding further up the descending colon, if you wish, for deeper cleansing. Another exercise you can add is the yogic abdominal lift. This exercise activates and stimulates the lower abdomen. Refer to your yoga book. (See resources section in appendix.)

Incidents of problems with colonics and enemas are rare and only occur in extreme cases from negligence and abuse. Driving a car is also dangerous and there are users who are reckless and there certainly is danger involved. But good drivers, who follow the rules, are careful and apply common sense, enjoy the benefits of driving without hazard. You are not likely to experience problems if you study and follow the guidance of professionals. The benefits of these important detoxification techniques far outweigh the minimal risks.

Daily Elements of a Fast

Cleansing
  Enema. Daily, every other day, or every third day.
  Colonic. Weekly or twice weekly.
Massage
  By a professional
  Self-massage with loofa skin brush
Walking
  Sunshine
  Air bath exposing skin as much as possible
Bath
  Steam bath at the health spa
  Epsom salt with tub bath
Dietary Intake
  Water
  Juice
  Herb Tea
  Hot Lemonade
Exercise
  Deep Breathing
  Yoga
  Walking
Rest
  Meditation
  Naps
  Deep Sleep

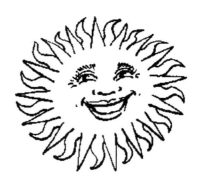

LOSING WEIGHT

Advantages of Fasting

The Europeans have an easy way of telling who is American. They just pick out the fat tourists! One out of 5 of us is overweight. That is 90 million Americans, and it is not because we have not been trying. There are literally thousands of specialized weight reduction diets. The bookstores and magazine ads are full of them. But what of it? No one method has the acclaim of universal and lasting success.

How unfortunate, because fasting could be that one method if it was not frowned upon as unorthodox and radical. When it comes to losing weight, fasting has no equal. Results are dramatic and lasting. Not only that, it is completely natural and superior to pills and drugs and all their unwanted side effects. The only side effects you get with fasting is a drop in high blood pressure along with the pounds.

How It Works

In order for the body to continue supplying energy during fasting, it utilizes its reserves in inverse order of importance. It takes fat (adipose) tissue first and vital muscle tissue from organs and glands last. In the obese, this can be as much as 65% of the total body weight. These people are best able to handle fasting for a long term once they get past the initial break-in period. When fat resources are depleted, true hunger returns and it is time to start eating.

What Can You Expect?

Overweight people can expect the greatest loss during the first week. The heavier you are, the more you will lose. This reward compensates for the difficulty of fasting, which is initially hard for most overweight people. After that, loss gradually tapers off in the following weeks until it stabilizes. Thinner people, of course, lose less. You may not loose as much as you wish, but it is probably all your body wants to release at this time. Whenever hunger returns, start eating.

Of course, this scenario will vary. Metabolic rates differ from person to person and variations exist even in an individual's ability to utilize calories. Thus a meal that could be fully utilized in the body of one person might accumulate fat in another. But no other method compares with fasting for swift weight loss and detoxification at the same time. Anything you do to assist detoxification, also assists weight loss. For those who fast just to loose weight, better health is a side effect!

Fundamentally, obesity indicates a malfunction in metabolism and/or digestion. But no special diet or pill treats the endocrine system. The thyroid controls metabolism. The adrenals control the reabsorption of sodium from the kidneys causing water retention. The pancreas contributes to fat and carbohydrate digestion. Fasting reduces the burden on these ductless glands as well as pressure on the heart. It improves the combustion and digestion of calories in addition to the alleviation of diseases of affluence such as diabetes, hypertension, ulcers, anemia, asthma, etc. True, we are all born with certain predispositions and we must learn to live within the confines of our body type. But long term fasting can reset certain biological patterns and provide new opportunities for the overweight.

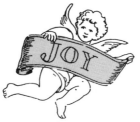

The Psychological Effects Of

FASTING

Are You Crazy?

Fasting is a very scary experience. The mere idea of not eating--not taking in food after a lifetime of daily meals--is an extraordinary idea. The challenge may understandably be frightening and you might question your wisdom in executing such a plan. There are physical issues here as well. Is not eating a question of life and death? Without food, won't we die? We eat so consistently, isn't it because we need to? What happens if we stop?

If these are some of the questions going through your mind, you could use a dose of outside support. But you won't get it! Fasting is a very lonely task. It is a form of unintended isolationism. After all, how can it be possible to move about and socialize in a world where all social events are oriented around food. People will feel for you, but they will try to persuade you to eat. Loved ones will be afraid for you. Medical people, who have little understanding of fasting, will bring the heavy weight of their positions of authority to bear on you in an attempt to broaden your insecurity and sabotage your foundation of strength.

When you started this fast you never expected to deal with other people's insecurities in addition to your own. But that is just the tip of the iceberg. When you fast, you are not just part crazy, you are an outcast. If you last, you will realize very soon that you are dealing with an eating world. Others may ridicule you or they may envy you. But it is the condemnation that will stick in your mind, not the praise. When you fast, you have to be firmly rooted in your conviction and in your confidence of what you are doing. That is why we discussed motivation. Motivation is your roots, which plant you firmly in the fast. Knowledge and guidance provide the strength and confidence to keep you from wavering in the winds of criticism and intimidation. If you are secure in what you are doing, you will soon realize that people are afraid of you and they are afraid of what you represent. You are making a statement by your actions for which some will admire and respect you. You may even become a mentor for some. But for others, you will reflect their own lack of courage and neglect for their bodies. You remind them of what they would rather not confront and they get angry as a cover for their insecurities. Their response is to condemn rather than face their own problems.

Keep A Diary

Fasting makes you an observer. It is like being in another time zone. You move to a different beat than the rest of the world. In fact, you might find yourself with too much time. After all, eating and sleeping take up lots of time and you will be doing less of both. It takes a little adjustment along with the physical adjustment that is involved in the early days.

Use your time productively. Monitor yourself: watch your appetite disappear. Observe your mind without its preoccupation with food. Watch the feeling of emptiness return to your gut. On long fasts, a diary is very important because it helps externalize your feelings as opposed to just storing an emotional memory of them. This is particularly important in regard to breaking the fast. When hunger first starts, it is subtle and can easily be ignored or confused with something else. There is a fine line between emotional/mental desire and physical hunger. Watch your attitude changes. Monitor any anger or resentment you may have about not eating. That is your signal to stop fasting. On the other hand, a positive attitude about the fast keeps you going for a long time. Your interest or disinterest in food is crucial to determining the length of your fast.

Fasting makes you an observer of yourself as well as others. When the experience is over, not only will you be changed, but you will also have an opportunity to help others break their bad habits. We are all victims of our own self-neglect. Help your fellow man/woman shed light on their fears. Turn their ignorance into knowledge and their knowledge will, in turn, help light the world.

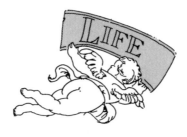

COMING OFF

THE FAST

Fasting is easy. It is the transition back to eating that is hard. When you are fasting you are "on a roll." Like a runner's high, once you get started, you can go (seemingly) forever. Discipline is not usually a factor during the fast, but it is required to start fasting and is the major factor in ending it.

Breaking The Fast

Anyone who is knowledgeable about fasting or who has had lots of experience will tell you that breaking the fast is the most important part. Willpower is required here, for once you engage your tastebuds and awaken your digestive secretions, it is as if you are waking a sleeping giant--and a hungry one, too! The hungry beast in you stirs quite quickly and is ready to ravage everything edible in sight. What's that? Not I, you say. Be forewarned: the desire for food is the strongest urge we have, and is even greater than the sexual drive!

Breaking the fast is both the hardest part of fasting and the most important. If you fail to restrain yourself from consuming too much--too soon, you will pay dearly for your errors. Pardon the dramatics, but this is also the most dangerous stage of the fast. You can hurt yourself here more than you could at any other time during the fast. Fatalities, few though they may be, occur while ending a fast. But do not worry. The statistics are in your favor and a fatal accident is highly unlikely. Nevertheless, you can get a whopper of a stomachache, one which might even send you to the hospital. The stress on your heart, liver, lungs and other vital organs could be so great as to undo the entire benefit of your fast. Of course, if you are only fasting for a few days, your transgressions will surely be survivable. But on a long fast, those of two weeks, 30 days or more, the shock to your system can provoke a heart attack in some cases. Even a short fast of three days can land you on your back with overwhelming nausea and a walloping belly ache if you are unable to curb your appetite.

Apologies are in order for the melodrama, but stories abound about fasters out of control, who break their fast with falafel, pizza, cookies and the like. You feel great while you are chewing: "Gee, this is just like old times. I can do this." After all, you are a pro at eating, it's true. But you are no longer a pro at digesting! And do not make the mistake of restraining yourself on the first day, then caving in on the second. Guaranteed, if you break your fast, even a relatively short one, with pizza, you will not be able to walk home.

Knowing When To Stop

Okay, melodrama over, but hold on, before we can discuss the proper way to break a fast, you have to know when to stop! In fact, choosing the right time to stop can make all the difference in breaking the fast. If you stretch yourself to make an "even two weeks," for example, or an "even month," you could be overextending yourself. After all, your body does not follow the calendar nor does it recognize your ego and your desires to "show off." If you stretch yourself beyond your needs, you can create a boomerang effect during the refeeding period and end up eating out of control.

The key: listen to your body. Recognize your interest in food when it occurs. Stop the fast when the desire for food returns. This happens slowly and subtly. It may first occur as an intellectual desire. You may find yourself asking questions about what is on your friend's plate. You may find yourself saying: "Mmm...that smells good!" Stop. Remember, when you are at the peak of your fast, no food interests you. It even smells repulsive.

Any intellectual change in your perspective is a forerunner of an actual desire for food. It is a signpost. You may also find yourself cheating in small ways, like taking in small amounts of pulp with your juice. Your desire to chew may return and you may find yourself chewing food, then spitting it out. All these are signposts. You may choose to ignore them at first, but take note. If they reoccur, go with them. It's time to eat! Use your fasting diary to help you monitor your feelings, then honor your feelings. If you ignore these signs, and let desire build up inside you, then the cravings will overwhelm and control you when you finally do start to eat. Knowing when to stop makes all the difference and allows you to complete your fast with self-control.

Real Hunger

Real hunger, by the way, is hard to ignore. When you get it, you will know it. If you ignore real hunger, then you are no longer fasting. You are starving. Starvation occurs when your body truly needs food and cannot get it. This is actually hard to do in today's world, unless you are on a desert island. But if, for example, you are on a political fast and refuse your body food, you will start to take nourishment from your muscles and organs. The starvation process draws from the least important tissues and organs first. In starvation, the body wants to build up and is seeking protein. In fasting, the body is cleansing and eliminating.

Timing

You may need to stop your fast because of your agenda. For example, if you are an actress and rehearsals are starting soon for a new play, you should schedule the breaking of your fast in time to build back your diet and full stamina. Or, if you have a wedding coming up that you must attend, it is necessary to allow sufficient time to build back your capacity to accommodate the excesses of a typical wedding feast. Don't wait until two days before! The temptations at such an occasion are overwhelming. Schedule the breaking of your fast with adequate time to rebuild your diet.

One final caution: Avoid ending your fast during a period of peak discomfort. A cleansing crisis may be taking place and it is wise to complete the process before reintroducing food. You may have a headache, a fever, nausea, sweats, a rash, etc. Generally, the rule is to wait until you feel better before you start eating.

The Road Back - Phase 1

Okay, so what's to eat? Fasts should be broken with soft, high water content foods. Usually, this means juicy fruits, but not necessarily. It could be a light soup, leafy green sprouts or a blended preparation. But before you even start to consider solid foods, begin by adding body to your juices. Now is the time to stop straining and add the sediment back to your juices. Mix in the powders such as spirulina, chlorella, and good tasting nutritional yeast. Enjoy nut milks made from almonds, sunflowers or sesame. These high protein, nutrient rich, powdered foods help to stimulate appetite and prepare your system for the heavier, solid foods. If these foods are satisfying, you can choose to extend your fast by consuming them for an additional day or two. Then, when you are ready, make the move to solid foods.

The most popular first food for breaking a fast is watermelon. Grapefruit is a close second. Oranges, grapes, apples, pears, pineapples and melons such as cantaloupe, crenshaw, papaya and mango are fine first foods. Peaches and apricots are a little heavier but can be taken at successive meals. The same is true for tomatoes (technically a fruit), cucumbers and green peppers, all high water content vegetables. If you have a desire for salads or vegetables early on, you can control your urges with green leafy sprouts and soup. Green sprouts such as alfalfa, clover, sunflower, buckwheat, turnip, cabbage, fenugreek, garlic, onion and radish are excellent. You can even use a small amount of alfalfa sprouts as your very first food to break your fast. First start with two or so individual sprouts then add more if comfortable. It is amazing how immensely satisfying a few sprouts are after a fast. Do not have "bean" sprouts such as mung, soy, lentil, adzuki, green peas, peanuts or garbanzos. These sprouts are too much like beans and require cooking and normal digestive strength.

Soups can be very satisfying, during the early meals, although you should not break a fast with them. Broths that were strained during the fast, can now be taken with the vegetable sediment. Miso paste can be added and if a desire for potatoes or grains exist, a light soup can be made as follows:

Cook rice with extra water. When the rice is
done, use the excess water as your soup base. You
may even leave 6 to 10 grains of rice in your base.
Next, add your vegetable broth mix, miso paste,
garlic, etc. Hot soup is very nourishing, and if you
want to make it hotter, add some cayenne pepper.
Cayenne stimulates circulation and strengthens the
stomach. A potato based soup can be made in the
same manner by boiling potatoes and using the
broth for your base. Blend a small chunk of potato
back into the water to strengthen the base. As each
day passes, you may blend larger amounts of potato
and larger amounts of rice, as long as your
stomach is not sending you a gurgling message to
stop.

So far, bananas have been missing from our menu. Banana is usually avoided during the early meals because it is a low water, high starch content fruit. It is especially starchy if taken unripe. Wait till your bananas become a rich yellow in color--better yet with brown spots--and blend with apple juice. Now we are increasing the water content of the meal. Start with half a banana and build up. If you enjoy this smoothie but want to chew, wait a few meals, then chew the banana again starting with half.

Smoothies can provide a whole menu of possibilities for the first or second day eater. Slippery elm, flax seed and chia all can be added to the banana-apple juice blend making a thicker and tastier drink. In addition, slippery elm is soothing to any inflammations in the stomach or digestive tract and chia and flax help restart peristaltic activity in the bowel. All create a mucilage or gel and have a nutty flavor as well as lots of nutrition.

Another food missing from the menu is dried fruit. Dried fruit has very little water content and is high in hard-to-digest fiber and sugar. However, certain dried fruits are soft and easy to digest when reconstituted. Figs, raisins, currants and prunes are excellent in reconstituted form, after the first day or two of feeding.

TYPICAL BREAKING AND EARLY FOODS

Fruits	Smoothies	
Watermelon	Banana	
Papaya	Apple	
Grapefruit	Chia	
Orange	Yeast	
Apple	Sunflower	
Peach	Sesame	
Pineapple	Slippery elm	
Cantaloupe	Psyllium	
Mango	Flax	
Other Melons	Spirulina	
Grapes	Chlorella	

Sprouts	Soups	Veggies
Alfalfa	Miso	Tomato
Clover	Broth	Cucumber
Buckwheat	Potato	Sw. Pepper
Sunflower		
Fenugreek		
Chia		

Quantity And Manner

Quantity and manner of consumption are vitally important. You can tolerate a wide variety of foods and indulge in minor transgressions, if taken in small amounts. Remember, your stomach is asleep. The glands that produce the digestive juices are relaxed and, in a manner of speaking, out of production. In fact, during the time you have not been eating, your stomach has shrunk! How much you eat and how you eat it is critical at this time. You can wake the sleeping giant with a crash, or with the smell of a rose.

First make sure you are sitting down when you eat. Digestion does not work as well when you are standing or in motion. Secondly, do everything slowly and conscientiously. Chew your juice. Sip your soup. The first meals should be taken like nectar from the gods. Afterwards, rest or recline keeping the head and shoulders higher than the stomach. Rest at first sign of tiredness. Never rush the refeeding process. Restrain yourself from becoming anxious or impatient. Do not push your body to return to full energy. Moderate your reinvolvement in physical activity. Remember, even though you have started eating, at this early phase you are still perpetuating the cleansing process started by the fast. This is the most important part of the whole fast. The manner in which you reintroduce food becomes more critical the longer you have fasted. As your taste sensations start to return, watch your quantities. Do not let your anxiety to eat or business plans overtake you. Listen to your stomach. If you hear gurgling or have gas, take it as a sign to slow down or eat smaller meals.

Priming The Pump

Turning on the glands is a gradual process. The key word here is: Nibble. Feed yourself like a baby. Take tiny amounts regularly every hour or two. Put yourself on a schedule and follow it. A half grapefruit at 8 a.m., an orange at 9:30, an apple at 11, a smoothie at 12, etc. Design a menu for the whole day and the next. Keep to it. Do not forget to have plenty of water in between and even a vegetable juice. Stick to the simple foods and avoid combinations. Each little bite sends signals through your nervous system stimulating the flow of digestive enzymes. Even if you choose to stay on a mono-diet, it is okay. Just take your apples, for example, regularly and in increasingly larger amounts.

You can also stimulate the digestive glands with herbs such as cinnamon and peppermint or seeds such as cloves and caraway. A honey vinegar drink helps stimulate the secretion of hydrochloric acid. Take 1 tablespoon of honey and 2 tablespoons of apple cider vinegar. Dilute with water to your tastes and drink before meals. Take some deep breaths before you start eating to add oxygen to your cells and stretch to awaken your whole body.

Foods and Supplements That Stimulate the Digestive System

Cinnamon	*Cardamon*
Peppermint	*Fennel*
Licorice	*Celery*
Star Anise	*Honey Vinegar*
Caraway	*HCL supplements*
Cloves	*Enzyme supplements*
Ginger	

What Is Phase I?

Phase I refers to the initial period after the fast where food is taken for the very first time. Here, the main task is to restimulate the digestive organs to the point where they can digest reasonably modest amounts of food. Soft, low density, high water content foods such as fruits, a few selected vegetables, sprouts, light soups and protein powder smoothies are used. The time required to build back the digestive system can take from one day to a week depending on the length of the fast and is represented by soft, easy to digest, high water content foods. On a 10 day fast, for example, the first post-fasting 5 days would be considered *phase I*. Days 6 through 10 would be *phase II* where a regime of denser foods would be followed. Days 11 through 15 is the post refeeding period where eating is largely returned to normal.

Phase II - Broadening The Meal Plan

Phase II starts with the premise that the digestive system has been turned back on and reasonable quantities of light foods can be consumed. The task of the *phase II* meal plan is to expand the dietary regime to include more complex and varied foods. *Phase I* builds on quantity. *Phase II* builds on variety. *Phase II* makes the transition from the cleansing cycle started by the fast to the building cycle--catabolic to anabolic. But this too, takes time and must be accomplished gradually. For the most part, once you have arrived at *phase II*, you are "out of the woods." From this point on, it is unlikely that any serious damage can be done to your digestive system or general health by eating the wrong foods. However, this is not to excuse wrong eating habits. You can still get terrible gas pains and ruin the overall positive effects of the fast by cheating at this point.

The predominant food during this phase is the salad. Green leafy vegetables and sprouts dominate. Fats are introduced in *phase II*, but only in the form of olives, olive oil, avocado and nuts and seeds and even so, not at the beginning. Tomatoes, olives, olive oil and lemon dressing, tamari, and later dressings made from sesame seeds, sunflower, tofu and avocado are some of the foods you can enjoy. But to start with, the first salad should be dry--without dressing.

Fruits are still a part of *phase II* but with no restrictions on quantity and variety. Dried fruits can now be consumed without reconstituting, however, some restriction on quantity should be maintained because of their high sugar and fiber content.

Nuts and seeds can be enjoyed in small quantities here. Use almonds and sunflower seeds as a condiment on salads or blend in smoothies or dressings.

Soups can be thicker with more vegetables and slightly higher amounts of blended rice or potato in the stock. Sea vegetables such as hijiki, dulse or kelp can be taken in the soups or as part of the salads.

The *phase II* regime is broader and more liberal, but it has its restrictions, too. No cooked vegetables (other than in soups), no grains or beans, including bread, and no dairy or animal products. These foods would be a part of *phase III* or days 11 through 15 in our example of a 10 day fast.

Phase II Foods

Spinach	*Dulse*	*Sesame seeds*
Lettuces	*Kelp*	*Sunflower*
Tomato	*Hijiki*	*Tofu*
Olive	*Condiments*	*Dried Fruit*
Avocado	*Olive Oil*	*Veget. Soups*
Sprouts	*Almonds*	*Phase I Foods*

Phase III - Transition Back To A Full Diet

Phase III basically signifies the beginning of the end of the fasting and refeeding period. However, if guidelines are followed, one can extend the benefits of the fast and avoid a quick return to the harmful dietary habits that prompted the fast in the first place.

Phase III starts the resumption of grains, starchy vegetables and cooked foods. Now is when you can sit down and have a bowl of rice or a baked potato. Steamed veggies like broccoli, string beans, zucchini, bean sprouts, etc. are some of the foods you can enjoy. There are no restrictions on dried fruits and nuts except those dictated by your own good judgment. Breads and cereal grains are fully available to you. Dairy and animal products can be consumed again, although we trust, judiciously. Remember, dairy and high fat foods are clogging to the digestive system. Deep fried foods like french fries should be avoided and high fat cheeses should be taken in moderation. Foods with added sugar should be kept to a minimum and foods with artificial and chemical agents, such as flavoring and dyes, should be avoided. The hard work and many wonderful benefits of your fast can be easily and quickly reversed if bad dietary practices are repeated.

Those Who Should Not Fast

Fasting is great, but not everyone should do it. Fasting puts the body in a cleansing and eliminating cycle. It shuts down many physiological processes for a usually well deserved rest. But those circumstances may not fit every person's needs and every situation.

Here are some people who should not fast:

Pregnant women
Nursing moms
Growing children
Most elderly
Most hypoglycemics
Diabetics

Those who are:
Critically ill
On long term medication
Underweight
Have tuberculosis
Advanced heart disease
Kidney dysfunction

Of course, there are always exceptions even with the above. But if you are uncertain, consult a health professional who knows fasting. Professional supervision should be mandatory before undertaking a fast with any of the above conditions. Hypoglycemics, for example, could benefit tremendously from a fasting or juice diet. But because their blood sugar and thus energy level drops dramatically when not eating, professional supervision is necessary.

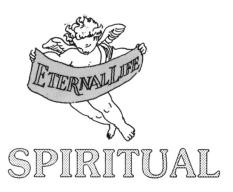

SPIRITUAL

FASTING

Fasting has been said to do more than just heal the body. It heals the soul. It restores harmony between the psyche and body and attunes the individual to his purpose and environment. When your body starts to heal, it is a spiritual experience, indeed, a miracle. You are at once initiated into the secrets of nature. When the body becomes clean, the mind becomes clear. You are reminded of your connection to your fellow human beings, the planet and the universe. It is an enlightening experience. Herbert Shelton, the father of fasting, said: the "freedom and ease you experience during abstinence enables you to discover new undreamed of depths to the meaning of life."

Religious people from all paths include fasting in their practices. Hindus and Jews, two of the most ancient religious groups, uphold the importance of fast days in the observance of certain religious holidays. They abstain not only from food, but from work. During the month of Ramadan, Muslims consume no food or drink between sunrise and

sunset. These faiths have as part of their theology the belief
that fasting benefits both the body and the soul and brings
disciples closer to God /Krishna /Allah.

Yogi's believe the body is the temple in which you live
and strive to keep it pure through proper diet, cleansing
techniques, hatha yoga exercises and periodic fasting. Christ-
ianity also has roots that acknowledge fasting. Jesus, in his
words taken from the *Essene Gospel of Peace*, advised his
followers to purify themselves.

> Purify, therefore, the temple that the Lord of the
> temple may dwell therein and occupy a place that
> is worthy of him. Renew yourselves and fast. For I
> tell you truly, that Satan and his plagues may only
> be cast out by fasting and by prayer. Go by yourself
> and fast anon, and show your fasting to no man.
> The living God shall see it and great shall be your
> reward. And fast till Beelzebub and all his evils
> depart from you and all the angels of our Earthly
> Mother come and see you. For I tell you truly, ex-
> cept you fast, you shall never be freed from the
> power of Satan and from all diseases that come
> from Satan. Fast and pray fervently, seeking the
> power of the living God for your healing.

True spiritual fasting is like a meditation. Ideally, it is
practiced in silence--no eating, no talking. You are alone
with your thoughts and eventually, at the point of total
peace, even they evaporate. Diet is not the issue. Weight is
not the issue. Discipline, spiritual growth and expansion of
consciousness is everything. Food connects you to your body
and the earth. Fasting releases your spirituality. You may
even discover some psychic abilities as waste products from

undigested food and other materials no longer interfere with nerve linkages and your vital energies are free to center in your upper chakras (energy centers) instead of your stomach. Conquering your appetite and desires allows you to focus your thoughts on the discovery of the 'heaven' within.

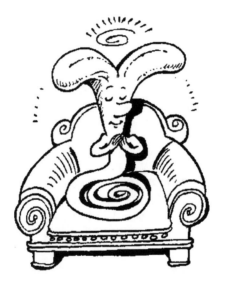

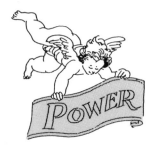

The Power
That Made The Body Can
HEAL
The Body

*The head is clearer, the health is better, the
heart is lighter and the purse is heavier.*
Scottish clergyman, circa 1800.

If these words were not known to be spoken by a Scottish clergyman some 200 years ago, they might be construed as a reference to a drug or utopian society. Unfortunately, fasting would be more popular if it was a drug. Imagine a pill that gives you the power to heal yourself. One that cleanses and strengthens your body, freshens your soul and renews your spirit? Such a pill would sell at any price. Ironically, fasting does not "sell" even though it is free. Yet, what a sublime and powerful tool we harbor inside us! Even more than a tool, it is a capacity, a power that is at our disposal at any time. To activate it--just stop eating. It is simple and effective, yet because of ignorance, fear, and lack of discipline, we let this power lie dormant most of our lives. How sad. We carry this "force" within us, but neglect to use it.

Why? Fasting takes courage. It requires will power, confidence and knowledge. These values are the fuel for your journey into fasting. Fasting means taking your health into your own hands. This is scary to most people and therefore courage and fortitude is required to begin. In truth, it is not always easy to do, but, for the most part, it is very easy to do. In fact, it is easier to fast than to eat and, ironically, it is more nutritious!

Juice fasting, the type of fasting we have been discussing, provides higher, more concentrated amounts of vitamins and minerals than solid food, and enables a higher percentage of assimilation. Thus, your cells actually receive more nourishment from juices than from food. After all, what is important is not how much you consume, but how much you utilize of what you take in. The vitamins, minerals, enzymes, live proteins, DNA and RNA hormones, and other mysteries of nature are all there in the fruits and vegetables. Unfortunately, our digestive systems are so inefficient that usually more nutrients are evacuated than assimilated. Clogged digestive tracts, inefficient organs and an over burdened digestive system reduce our ability to assimilate the food we eat. On the other hand, when you drink juice, you bypass the early sections of the digestive tract so even those with weak digestion are able to absorb 95+% of the nutrition that is there. Raw juices provide "pre-digested" microscopic nutrients that cells and tissues require. In fact, there is more nutrition in any green vegetable juice than in a plate of salad. It's concentrated! While you could never consume a pound of carrots, you can easily drink a glass of juice made from a pound of carrots (approximately 10½ ounces). You get its nourishment faster and more of it. Juice fasting is the closest thing to a transfusion without an injection!

As if this were not enough, every study in longevity shows that frugal eating promotes health and prolongs life. What you miss in the pleasures of eating, you make up for in the joys of living and feeling great. Fast and you sharpen your wits, increase your feeling of youthfulness, radiate natural beauty, become aware of your own spirituality and attunement to higher vibrations. We really need fasting in today's world. One cannot continue to live in any fast paced, high stressed, overindulgent, demanding lifestyle without availing his/her body and mind of an opportunity to rest. Sleep cannot always provide this. The multiplicity of dreams, nightmares, fears and neuroses are proof. The body must unwind and recover with its own physiological vacation.

Ironically, it is fear that keeps us from fasting. We are afraid if we halt the familiar routine of feeding our bodies, we will starve or become unwell. Those who are ignorant of fasting equate it with starving. Astounding though it may seem, the human body can live without food for an incredibly long time. In fact, instead of feeling weak and ill, you may very well feel more energetic. It is a paradox, but fasting creates efficiency. The aphorism: "to get more done, slow down," holds true here, too. In fasting, it is "to eat more, eat less." After fasting, the digestive tract is cleansed and better able to assimilate nutrients once eating is resumed.

Of course, there is good fasting and bad fasting. Like our friend who broke his fast with falafel, you can make a mess of it. Education is absolutely necessary. Start slowly with a short fast to get your feet wet and build your confidence, or, make sure you have professional guidance. Confidence is crucial when fasting. It can mean the difference between an easy fast and one filled with fears. Study. Go to lectures. Listen to audio tapes. Seek counseling. Talk to others more experienced than you. Get to know local people in the movement and read, read, read. Ultimately, fasting is a very personal experience and the full experience can only be acquired by actual involvement. This is the most powerful of all tools for cleansing which is at your disposal at any time if you know how to use it.

Ideally, fasting should be a custom that is part of our culture. Everybody should fast (apart from the exceptions on p.116.) just as everyone should clean their house. Ironically, it is often the people who keep their homes meticulously clean, that are guilty of neglecting their bodies. The Yogis think of the body as their temple. How much better our national health would be if we cleaned our bodies once a week like we clean our houses. A one day fast every week is a gift of fresh air and relaxation for the body. It amounts to 50 days off a year. Such a simple technique can actually extend your life! We are very well focused on cleaning our homes, whether it is once a week, once a month, spring cleaning, winter cleaning, raking leaves, mowing the lawn, dusting, polishing, covering with plastic, etc. What great care we give it! If only we could direct some of that fastidiousness to our *internal* homes. Perhaps, we should think of it as a business arrangement. Fasting is a small investment that pays you back a thousand fold. It is physical insurance. The only startup costs are the elimination of fear and ignorance.

Although we are discussing fasting, the real issue here is health. Fasting is the method. Health is the goal. The philosophy promulgated here is simple: eat well, live right and respect your body. So when you have fasted and it is all done, remember the philosophy. As wonderful as fasting is, it is not a magic wand, and a short fast a long time ago is meaningless to your health today. Make fasting a part of your total health program, which should include proper diet, exercise, rest, clean air, water and sunshine, as well as the elimination of bad habits such as smoking, bingeing, excess sugar, alcohol, coffee, etc. If these concepts of better health fit your philosophy, then discover fasting. Fast and your mind becomes clearer, your mental attitude improves and your self-esteem is enhanced. Each day you awake feeling younger and stronger. It is a gift and it is available right now. Give yourself that gift. Take the *Fast* way to health.

REVIEW
Basic Principles of Fasting

Motivation: Reasons to Fast
Detoxification
Weight Loss
Healing
Spiritual
Break Addictions
Political/Social
Dental Work

Conditions Fasting Has Helped

Allergies	Acne
Asthma	Rheumatism
Hay Fever	Ulcers
Hives	Liver Problems
Migraines	Gall Stones
Obesity	Constipation
Insomnia	Diarrhea
High and Low Blood Pressure	

Criteria for Choosing the Length of the Fast
Fasting Experience
Physical Strength & Condition
Nature of Illness, if any
Previous Diet, Level of Toxicity
Age, Mental Attitude
Schedule of Work and Activities
Environment and Weather

Prerequisites for Water Fasting

Experience or Professional Guidance
Aversion to Juices and other Liquids
Lots of Rest. No Stress Environment
Keep to yourself. Silence if possible
Avoidance of TV and Radio
Do yoga or gentle stretching
Bathe in the Sun and in Mineral waters
Lay on the Grass. Meditate
Fresh, Clean Air, Warm Weather
Read Fasting, Health or Spiritual books

What to Mix in Your Fruit & Vegetable Juices

CARROT JUICE	GREEN JUICE	FRUIT JUICE
Carrot	Celery	Pineapple
Beet	Spinach	Orange
Green Pepper	Tomato	Grapefruit
Cucumber	Cabbage	Watermelon
Alfalfa	Dill	Apple
Watermelon Rind	Lemon	Pear
Apple	Garlic	Grape
Ginger	Cayenne	

Other Non–Juice Drinks

Some of these recipes must be strained and used sparingly
Almond, Sesame and Sunflower Nut Milks
Vegetable Soup Broths
Wheatgrass Juice
Chlorophyll Powders mixed with juice such as Spirulina, Chlorella or Blue-Green Algae
Nutritional Yeast
Psyllium Colon Cleanser
Homozone Colon Oxygenator

Herb Teas for Digestion

Peppermint	Spearmint	Licorice
Cinnamon	Ginger	Burdock

Food Color And Its Healing Effects

Red	Circulation
Orange	Anti-spasmodic
Yellow	Nerves
Green	Blood Purifier
Blue	Spiritual/Mental

Detoxification Techniques

Massage
Air Brushing
Bath of Epsom Salt
Steam Bath
Colonics, Enemas
Psyllium Seed or Flax Seed Bulk Laxative Drinks
Exercise

Organs of Elimination

Lungs
Skin
Kidneys
Eyes
Liver
Colon
Tongue

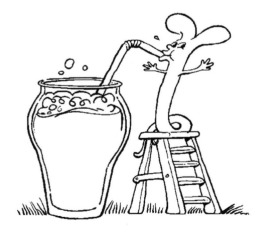

Symptoms of a Healing Event

Rash	Headache
Eczema	Faintness
Acne	Fever
Nausea	Diarrhea
Weakness	Muscle Aches
Dizziness	Bad Breath
Hot Flashes	Stuffed Nose
Fatigue	Running Nose
Bronchitis	Irregular Heartbeat
Asthma	Irregular Menstruation

Fasting Exercises

Yoga	Aerobics	Biking
Walking	Swimming	Trampolining
	Deep Breathing	

Signals Telling You When to Stop the Fast
Applicable to fasts one week or longer

Desire for Food
Curiosity about what others are Eating
Desire to Chew
Attraction to Aromas
Busy or Stressful Personal Schedule
Desire for Protein
Desire for Heavier, richer drinks
Cravings
Real Hunger

HOW TO BUY A JUICER

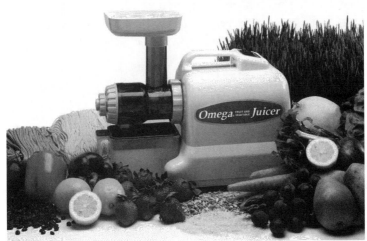

Whether you are fasting or not, a fruit and vegetable juicer can become the most important nutritional appliance in your home. As a dispenser of vitamins and minerals alone, you will find this machine provides hundreds of dollars of savings worth of store-bought supplements each year. And that does not count all the fun you and your family will have in using it. It is a magic thirst quenching machine that conjures all kinds of flavors and colors to interest even the most soda-pop minded family members. If you're a health-seeker, it is your personal drug store and medicine chest for all that ails you.

Good juicers generally range in price from $125–$300 with, of course, exceptions. The under $125 machines are often products of large appliance manufacturers such as Sunbeam, GE, Westinghouse, and Sanyo, to name a few, that make a full line of kitchen products and/or other appliances. Some companies, like Sanyo and Sony for example, are known mostly for their radio equipment, but have expanded into juicers to take advantage of their popularity. Many of these products are multi-purpose machines that also blend, whip and process, as well as juice. This is in contrast to a 'dedicated' machine which only juices. The multipurpose appliances are invariably the poorest juicers. As a general caveat, if it dices, slices and plays in stereo, avoid it.

Different Juicing Systems

Centrifugal Force   Twin Gear
Trituration   Worm Gear

In regard to the extraction of nutrients, four different kinds of juicing systems are available. The first of these is commonly known as 'centrifugal' because it uses centrifugal force. Vegetables cut into tiny pieces are spun around in a basket at high speed (3,000–7,000 rpm's) and the juice is extracted by the sheer power of centrifugal force. This is the same way wet clothes are relieved of their excess water in a washing machine during the spin cycle. This is the basic principle of centrifugal force. The second method is known as 'trituration' and operates by chewing and ripping the vegetables up and then forcing the ripped pulp against a screen with the pressure of the rotating cutter. The triturator operates at a slower speed (1,750 rpm's) and has much less exposure to air. It doesn't whip anything around. Because the high speed spinning of centrifugal juicers creates greater oxidation (destruction of nutrients), triturators have higher nutritional ratings. Another significant difference involves the way each machine cuts. Triturators rip into the vegetable with fairly dull teeth, while centrifugal machines cut them into pieces using sharp blades. The ripping process is purported to break open the plant membranes exposing nutrients and enzymes for extraction. The blades of a centrifugal juicer slice the vegetables into tiny pieces that, at least theoretically, do not penetrate as deep. This is the controversial but essential difference between the two methods.

The Mail Order Catalog carries the full line of books published by Book Publishing Company, plus many other alternative presses.

If you are interested in other fine books on vegetarian cooking, alternative health, or Native Americans, please mark your area of interest below and send for our catalog, or call 1-800-695-2241.

I would like to receive your book catalog on:

Vegetarian cooking and nutrition ☐

Alternative health ☐

Native Americans ☐

_____

Name

_____

Street or P.O. Box

_____

City   State   Zip

See our vegetarian & health titles on the web at:

www.healthy-eating.com

Another method is the old reliable worm gear. Many of these juicers are cast iron affairs similar to the old table top hand-crank meat grinders that were popular during the mid-century. These machines are good for fruits and leafy vegetables, but are primarily wheatgrass juicers. They come as manual or motorized machines and range in price from $100—$600. Even the motorized ones turn a gentle 100 rpm's which is ideal for protecting fragile nutrients.

The newest juicing system is the twin gear masticator. This patented technology is both innovative and unique. Two gears fold inwardly on each other, crushing the vegetables and forcing the juice out against a fine sieve. The gears' 90 rpm speed is as slow as if you were hand cranking it. This eliminates the heat caused by friction of the faster running machines as well as the oxidation that is exacerbated by the wind from the high velocity blades. Crushing or mastication is the best way to crack the plant's cell walls and reach deeply entrenched nutrients. These machines are also versatile in that they will juice wheatgrass in addition to common vegetables. Thus, if you ever want to explore the wonders of wheatgrass, you don't have to find space for two machines. They cost about $500.

What to Shop For

First, start by shopping for a dedicated juicer, that is a machine that is designed and promoted for juicing only. If it incidently performs other tasks, that is okay. Dedicated juicers are stronger, better designed and, indeed, cost more, than multifunction machines. When shopping for a juicer, consider the following criteria:

1. Capacity to Extract Nutrients	4. Size and space
	5. Price
2. Neatness & Convenience of operation	6. Warranty Term
	7. Motor Power
3. Efficiency of Clean-up	8. Pulp Disposal Method

When it comes to using a juicer, the convenience of operation and clean-up are probably the two major factors you will be dealing with on a day to day basis. If you are discouraged with the clean-up and set up of your juicer, you will probably stop using it. This is an even more important factor than its capacity for nutrient extraction. If you don't like to use your juicer, you won't get many nutrients, even from the most expensive machine. On the other hand, if you use and enjoy it every day, you will get lots of nutrition. Regular use is the secret to unleashing the power of juice therapy.

All machines have to be assembled and disassembled for use. They all have a cutter blade or gear, a cover, a screen and a housing or a juicer body to remove and clean. You can compare the differences in handling the parts of the different types of juicers ad infinitum. But they all have 3–5 parts you must clean and reassemble. In the end, the speed and efficiency of clean-up and reassembly is much about what you get used to.

The pulp-ejector machines expel the pulp continuously while the machine is juicing. This is a big time saver if you want to juice more than half a gallon at once. You don't have to stop juicing to clear out the pulp. Non-ejecting juicers collect the pulp in spinning baskets which must be emptied after juicing two quarts. This becomes an issue if you are juicing for the whole family or making a gallon of juice for your fast. On the plus side, many basket juicers come with optional paper filters that make clean-up easier, faster and neater.

Something to consider along with clean-up is ease of use. The triturators and masticating twin gears require more oomph to insert the carrots than centrifugal machines which literally gobble them up. Consider who is going to do the juicing and make the best match. The centrifugal machines, with their sharp blades, draw in the vegetables easily and at a faster rate. However, both types of machines are laborious when it comes to juicing greens. Leafy vegetables need to be alternated with watery fruits like tomatoes or cucumbers or stiff vegetables like carrots and beets. Put the spinach in first, then the tomato, spinach, cucumber, spinach, etc.

Finally, in considering which juicer to buy, we come to the practical decisions of size, space and price. This may settle it for you right here. Your budget is your budget and even though you may crave the more expensive machines, perhaps you should start small and upgrade slowly. On the other hand, you may not want a machine that is too big or too heavy. Remember, choosing which to buy, all boils down to how it will be used. Pick a machine that you will use and enjoy on a daily basis.

Can't Buy a Juicer?

If you do not have a juicer and cannot buy one now, you can fast primarily on non-juice drinks such as teas, broths, powdered juices, fresh apple cider and home made citrus juice. If you do not have a good citrus juicer, invest in one. Even the electric ones can be purchased for $10—$20 and they will serve you well.

Then, of course, there are always the juice bars. Many health food stores and juice bars offer freshly made vegetable and wheatgrass juice. With supplementation from your home citrus juicer and other non-juice drinks, you can still fast on a wide variety of vital drinks.

If you are really out in the woods, there is one other thing you can do. Purchase a fine stainless steel hand vegetable grater and grind your carrots down by hand. Place the grated carrot in a cheese cloth or sprout bag and squeeze. Twist the bag until juice pours out and catch it in a bowl. Messy? Maybe, but definitely delicious and all without electricity.

A Few Caveats

No matter what method you use, remember to strain your juice. Most juicers include filter papers or stainless steel strainers. Use them. Unstrained juice allows invisible particles of pulp to enter your stomach. While not a problem when eating, these small solids add up and stimulate the flow of digestive enzymes, making you hungry—not something you want on your fast!

Do not use your blender. Blenders make purees, not juices. True, the purees could be strained but this will not get you much nutrition, especially considering that high speed blenders tend to oxidize the juice and thereby devitalize it. Also avoid the temptation of bottled juices. These are boiled, sweet, flavored waters and are not alive with the nutrition you need.

Popular Juicing Machines

What follows is a list of some of the most popular dedicated juice machines available. This is in no way a complete list, however, these models are proven industry leaders and, in some cases, have been on the market for decades. Purchase them through your local natural food store, natural lifestyle catalog, the internet or see the resource section of this book for supplier and manufacturer names and numbers. Prices listed are the manufacturer's "suggested retail" prices as of 2002.

Omega Juicers

Omega is an international leader in juicing machines. They manufacture high quality centrifugal, worm–gear, and pulp ejector

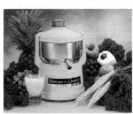

juicers. Their model 1000 is an industry standard. It is a stainless steel—bowl, basket, and blade—centrifugal juicer with a 2 quart capacity. It has a strong one-third h.p. G.E. motor rated at 250 watts, spins at 3,600rpm's, weighs 11 lbs. and comes with a fabulous 10 year warranty. This USA made

Omega 1000. A centrifuge.

machine also offers a citrus attachment and paper filters for easy and neat pulp collection. Priced under $250. Also investigate its pulp ejector brother, model 4000, that comes with an incredible 15 year warranty. Priced under $300.

The Omega model 8001—pictured on page 129—is one appliance that performs many kitchen chores. It will juice any produce including wheatgrass. Its low 80 revolutions per minute means less foam, no heat build up, no destruction of vitamins, and no oxidizing of the juice. It is as gentle to the food as an old fashioned hand crank. It is a single, worm-gear style machine that masticates the juice. This means it chews and breaks open vegetable fibers, releasing nutrients from deep within the cell walls. Because it is also a pulp ejector, it will continuously juice wheatgrass and vegetables and automatically eject the pulp.

When you are done juicing, start making almond butter, peanut butter, cashew butter, sunflower butter... and more. Then, freeze your extra bananas and churn them through the 8001 to make a creamy but dairy-free banana ice cream. Add blueberries, strawberries, raspberries, and extrude them all into unbelievable desserts. Baby foods, pastas, and differently shaped noodles are made with the extruding feature. Feed your baby from nature, not from a jar.

This is a powerful (2 horsepower), heavy duty machine, but is the quietest juicer around. The pulp is very, very dry and there are lots of creature features to make your juicing easier. You get a cleaning brush, food pusher, a generously sized hopper, a sieve, and different juicing nozzles and strainers, and a tight fitting collection bowl. All this makes for a neat, and convenient juicing experience. 5 year warranty. Priced under $350.

Miracle Exclusives

Miracle Exclusives is an importer of health oriented kitchen appliances with a full line of juicers, including manual and electric wheatgrass juicers and commercial juice bar models. Their Millennium juicer® model MJ2000 is a centrifugal, pulp ejecting juicer with

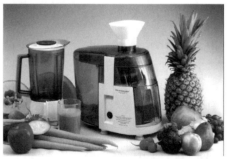

Miracle Millennium Juicer® is available with a Blender attachment for smoothies.

many high end features for a very affordable price. It boasts a 350 watt motor, a finely crafted stainless steel cutting blade and basket, a uniquely designed internal collection bottle, and an oversized external hopper which just pops off to empty. A blender attachment is available so you can make juices and smoothies with one machine for a non-stop flow of liquid vitamins. 3 year warranty. Price $175.

L'Equip

This new American company with the French sounding name premiered their L'Equip pulp ejector model 221 in 1999. It has striking looks and impressive state-of-the-art features including a servo-controlled 420 watt motor that constantly monitors and regulates the speed of the cutting blades according to the type of fruits and vegetables being juiced. The pulp ejector comes with a disposable catch-bag in addition to the traditional plastic bin for the ultimate in no-mess convenience. This centrifugal juicer has a stainless

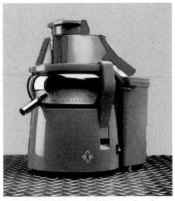

L'Equip 221 stainless steel pulp ejector with computerized motor speed control and 12 year warranty.

steel bowl, blade, and basket and an amazing 12 year warranty. Price under $250. In 2001, they premiered a smaller "mini" version of this model which has nearly the same features but is about half the price.

Champion Juicer

This is arguably the oldest juicer in the USA market. It is a pulp ejecting triturator which means it grinds and crushes rather than cuts the vegetables. The blade's teeth are stainless steel as well as the internal juicer housing. This versatile machine also grinds nuts and seeds into nut butter and makes delicious frozen fruit sherbert. An attachment for grinding grains into flour is also available. The Champion is a heavy duty machine with a 1/3 hp motor that turns at a moderate 1,725rpm's. 5 year warranty. Made in USA. Under $300.

Green Power

This company introduced the innovative, triturating twin gear system into the USA market in 1994. Not only was it innovative and unique, it was also avant-garde. Inside the twin stainless steel gears are magnets and ceramics that produce positive ions as the gears spin. According to the designers, this effect results in less oxidation and greater longevity of the fresh juice. The company provides the results of an independent lab study evaluating carrot and apple juice over 72 hours.

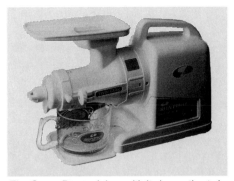

The Green Power Juicer with its innovative twin gear design was the first affordable machine to juice wheatgrass along with regular vegetables.

Theoretically, the juice lasts longer because more enzymes and nutrients are kept intact, enhancing stability.

This is a versatile machine that will juice carrots and wheatgrass at the same time. Traditionally, these two required different juicing machines. Juicing carrots right along with your wheatgrass is wonderful for both taste and convenience and may convert even the most reluctant wheatgrass drinkers. Use this same machine to entertain non-wheatgrass guests with nut butters, frozen fruit sorbets, mochi (Japanese rice cakes) and 3 different shapes of pasta.

The twin gears turn at a slow 110rpm's, crushing the vegetables and forcing the juice out against a fine sieve. Since it is also a pulp ejector, you can juice continuously without stopping to clean. When you do need to clean up, there are four parts to wash and remount: the twin gears, strainer and front and back housing. This is no more or less than setting up and cleaning a common vegetable juicer. It also comes with a sturdy built-in handle for moving and storing. No surprise it won the 1993 Silver medal prize in Germany at the International Exhibition of Inventions. The *Green Star juicer* comes with a two year warranty. Priced under $550.

See the Resources chapter to get contact information for juicer manufacturers and distributors.

RESOURCES

Where to Go to Get more Help and Information

Healing Resorts that Juice & Fast

The Tree of Life Rejuvenation Center. PO Box 1080, Patagonia, Arizona, 85624. 520-394-2520, fax 415-598-2409. www.treeoflife.nu A spiritual, mountain retreat directed by renowned holistic physician and author, Gabriel Cousens, M.D. Their "planetary healing" approach includes fresh juice fasting, detoxification, meditation, yoga, sprouts, wheatgrass, and live-food Kosher cuisine.

Regency Health Spa. 2000 So. Ocean Dr., Hallandale, FL 33009. 800-454-0003, 954-454-2220. Dr. Frank Sabatino supervises raw juice and water fasting in this gourmet vegetarian health spa that emphasizes weight loss, nutrition, stress management and personal fitness. www.RegencyHealthSpa.com

Hallelujah Acres. 800-651-7622, tel: 704-481-1700, fax: 704-481-0345, PO Box 2388, Shelby, NC 28151 www.HAcres.com. In Canada www.HAcres.com/Canada. A religious, spiritual, raw foods and fasting retreat center founded by the Rev. Paul Malkmus.

Ann Wigmore Institute - Puerto Rico. PO Box 429, Rincon, PR 00677. 787-868-6307, 787-868-0591. www.AnnWigmore.org

New Age Health Spa. Neversink, NY 12765. 845-985-7601. Beautiful Catskill mountain spa offering juice fasting weeks. www.NewAgeHealthspa.com

Hippocrates Health Centre of Australia. [61] 75-530-2860. Mudgeeraba Queensland, Australia. www.hippocrates.com.au

We Care. 18000 Long Canyon Road, Desert Hot Springs, CA 92241. 800-888-2523. 760-251-2261, fax: 760-251-5399 www.WeCareSpa.com Rejuvenation and detoxification program at secluded ranch in California desert.

TrueNorth Health Center. 4310 Lichau Road, Penngrove, CA 94951. Tel. 707-586-5555. www.healthpromoting.com Offering both residential and outpatient therapeutic fasting guided by a team of medical, chiropractic, and psychology doctors.

Optimum Health Institute - San Diego. 800-993-4325.
619-464-3346, fax 619-589-4098. www.optimumhealth.org
Wheatgrass, raw juices, detoxification, living foods health program.

Optimum Health Institute - Austin, Texas. 800-993-4325,
512-303-4817, fax 512-303-1239. Wheatgrass, raw juices,
detoxification, living foods health program. www.optimumhealth.org

Hippocrates Health Institute - West Palm Beach, Florida.
561-471-8876, fax: 561-471-9464. Wheatgrass, raw juices,
detoxification, living foods health program. www.hippocratesinst.com

Tanglewood Wellness Center. Thurmont, MD. 301-898-8901.
www.TanglewoodWellnessCenter.com. Mountaintop retreat center for
supervised water fasting one hour from Washington, DC.

More Information & Help

Sproutman. The author offers guided fasting and telephone
consultations on related health and diet issues. 413-528-5200, fax 413-
528-5201. Sproutman@Sproutman.com   www.Sproutman.com

Fasting Center International. Dennis Paulson. Santa Barbara,
CA 93101. 805-899-4998, Fax 805-962-5988. www.Fasting.com
Telephone and internet juice fast guidance by the master faster.

Preventive Medical Center of Marin. 25 Mitchell Blvd #8, San
Rafael, CA 94903. 415-472-2343, Fax 415-472-7636. Elson M Haas,
MD author of *The Detox Diet* guides clients on fasting and
detoxification programs. www.ElsonHaas.com

Rhio's Raw Energy Hotline. 212-343-1152. Living foods help
line and resource directory of classes and events in the New York
metro area and beyond. www.RawFoodInfo.com

San Francisco Live Food Enthusiasts. The *Sproutline* 415-751-
2806. Telephone help line and listing of live foods pot-lucks, lectures
and outings in the San Francisco region.

RawTimes. An extensive website resource of testimonials, e-mail
forums, recipes, restaurant reviews, networking, events, and book
reviews on living foods diet. www.rawtimes.com

American Holistic Health Association. P.O. Box 17400, Anaheim, CA 92817-7400. 714-779-6152. www.ahha.org Resource lists for holistic practitioners and healing centers.

International Association for Colon Hydrotherapy. San Antonio, TX 78230. 210-366-2888, Fax 210-366-2999. www.i-act.org Find a colon hydrotherapist near to you.

American Natural Hygiene Society. PO Box 30630, Tampa, FL 33630. 813-855-6607. Founded by Herbert Shelton, father of water fasting. Magazine and annual convention. www.anhs.org

Manufacturers of Fasting Related Products

Healthy-Eating Catalog. Summertown, Tenn. 800-695-2241, fax 931-964-2291. www.Healthy-Eating.com Sells Sproutman's Organic Sprouting Seeds, sprout bags, books, juicers, and vegan supplies.

Renew Life. Clearwater, FL 33765. 800-830-4778. 813-871-3200, fax 813-938-1155. Makers of colon cleansers and the Life-Step, for correct toilet posture. www.renewlife.com

Colema Boards. V.E. Irons, Inc. PO Box 2205, Kansas City, MO 64142. 800-544-8147. Fax 916-347-5921. Makers of Sonne, the original line of colon cleansers, the colema board, a home colonic unit and GreenLife grass powder. www.colema-boards.com

Green Foods Corporation 320 North Graves Ave, Oxnard, CA 93030. 800-777-4430, fax 805-983-8843. Makers of *Green Magma* barley grass juice plus carrot juice, wheat germ juice and vegetable juice powders. www.greenfoods.com

Pines International, Inc. PO Box 1107, Lawrence, KS 66044. 1-800-MY-PINES (800-697-4637), Fax 913-841-1252. Grass and beet juice powders. www.wheatgrass.com

Greens✝. Orange Peel Enterprises, Inc. 2183 Ponce de Leon Circle, Vero Beach, FL 32960. 800-643-1210, fax 561-562-9848. www.greensplus.com First manufacturer of a multi-green, grasses, algae, etc., juice powder.

Kyo-Green. Wakunaga of America Co. Ltd. 23501 Madero, Mission Viegjo, CA 92691. 800-421-2998. 714-855-2776. Fax 714-458-2764. www.kyolic.com Japanese grown grass and chlorella juice powders.

Jamba Juice. 1700 Seventeenth Street, San Francisco, CA 94103. 415-865-1134, fax 415-487-1143. Largest of the national juice bar chains. Contact them to find a juice bar location near you.

Other Books on Juices and Fasting

Power Juices Super Drinks. *Quick, Delicious Recipes to Reverse and Prevent Disease* by Steve Meyerowitz. 424 pages. 2000. $14. Nutrition and health benefits of various fruits, vegetables, and herbs. Recipes for common ailments using juices, teas, and smoothies. For excerpts, table of contents, etc. visit www.Sproutman.com.

Wheatgrass Nature's Finest Medicine. *The Complete Guide to Using Grass Foods & Juices to Help Your Health* by Steve Meyerowitz. 1999. 216pg. $12.95. The latest nutrition information and research on the healing power of the different grass juices. For table of contents and excerpts visit, www.Sproutman.com

The Detox Diet. by Elson M Haas, MD. 1996. 128 pgs. ISBN# 0890878145. An excellent resource to maximize detoxification.

The Juiceman's Power of Juicing. by Jay Kordich, the original Juiceman! 1992. 286 pgs. ISBN #0688114431.

The Miracle of Fasting. By health pioneer Paul Bragg. $8.95

Fasting and Eating for Health. *A Medical Doctor's Program for Conquering Disease.* by Joel Fuhrman, M.D. 255pp. $15.

Fasting Can Save Your Life Video. Experiences shared by patients fasting at the TrueNorth Health Clinic (see "Resorts") and their doctors. Answers to many common questions. 68 minutes, $23.

Juicing for Life: *A Guide to the Health Benefits of Fresh Fruit and Vegetable Juicing* by Cherie Calbom & Maureen Keane. 1992.

Heinerman's Encyclopedia of Healing Juices by Dr. John Heinerman. 1996. 336 pgs Prentice Hall. ISBN #0130575712.

Juicer Manufacturers & Distributors

Green Power Juicer - Tribest, Inc. 888-254-7336, fax 562-623-7160. Santa Fe Springs, CA 90670 www.greenpower.com

Miracle Exclusives, Inc. PO Box 8, Port Washington, NY 11050. 800-645-6360, fax 516-621-1997. www.MiracleExclusives.com

Omega Juicers. 800-633-3401, fax 717-561-1298. PO Box 4523, Harrisburg, PA 17111. www.Omegajuicers.com

L'Equip. 555 Bolser Ave., Harrisburg, PA 17043. 800-816-6811. 717-730-7100, fax 717-730-7200. www.Lequip.com

Albion Enterprises. 3233 Coffee Lane #H, Santa Rosa, CA 95403. 800-248-1475. 707-528-1473, fax 707-528-0608. www.albionjuicer.com

ACME Equipment Co. 1024 Concert Ave. Springhill, FL 34609. 800-882-0157. fax 352-683-7740. www.AcmeEquipment.com

TJ Plus. 5631 East Morning Star Road, Cave Creek, AZ 85331. 888-243-6450. 602-488-7808, fax 602-488-7895. www.juicebars.com

Back To Basic Products. 11660 South State St. Draper, UT 84020-9455. 800-688-1989. 801-571-7349, fax 801-571-6061. www.Backtobasicproducts.com

HealthWise. 13659 Victory Blvd #525, Van Nuys, CA 91401. 800-942-3262. 818-942-3262, fax 818-982-1471. wwwHwhealth.com

INDEX